100 Questions & Answers About Chronic Obstructive Pulmonary Disease (COPD)

Campion E. Quinn, MD

JONES AND BARTLETT PUBLISHERS

Sudbury, Massachusetts

BOSTON   TORONTO   LONDON   SINGAPORE

World Headquarters
Jones and Bartlett Publishers
40 Tall Pine Drive
Sudbury, MA 01776
978-443-5000
info@jbpub.com
www.jbpub.com

Jones and Bartlett Publishers
Canada
6339 Ormindale Way
Mississauga, ON L5V 1J2
CANADA

Jones and Bartlett Publishers
International
Barb House, Barb Mews
London W6 7PA
UK

Jones and Bartlett's books and products are available through most bookstores and online booksellers. To contact Jones and Bartlett Publishers directly, call 800-832-0034, fax 978-443-8000, or visit ourwebsite www.jbpub.com.

Substantial discounts on bulk quantities of Jones and Bartlett's publications are available to corporations, professional associations, and other qualified organizations. For details and specific discount information, contact the special sales department at Jones and Bartlett via the above contact information or send an email to specialsales@jbpub.com.

Copyright © 2006 by Jones and Bartlett Publishers, Inc.

Library of Congress Cataloging-in-Publication Data
Quinn, Campion.
  100 questions & answers about chronic pulmonary obstructive disease
(COPD) / Campion E. Quinn.
    p. cm.
  ISBN 0-7637-3638-4 (pbk.)
    1. Lungs—Diseases, Obstructive—Miscellanea.   I. Title. II. Title:
100 questions and answers about chronic pulmonary obstructive disease
(COPD). III. Title: Questions & answers about chronic pulmonary
obstructive disease (COPD).
RC776.O3Q56 2006
616.2'4—dc22

                                    2005017242

Production Credits
Executive Publisher: Christopher Davis
Production Director: Amy Rose
Associate Production Editor: Kate Hennessy
Editorial Assistant: Kathy Richardson
Associate Marketing Manager: Laura Kavigian
Manufacturing and Inventory Coordinator: Therese Connell
Composition: Northeast Compositors
Cover Design: Kate Ternullo
Cover Images: Clockwise from left © Photodisc, © Thinkstock, © Pixtal/age fotostock
Printing and Binding: Malloy, Inc.
Cover Printing: Malloy, Inc.

Printed in the United States of America
09 08 07 06 05   10 9 8 7 6 5 4 3 2 1

For My Wife Nancy

Contents

Part 1: What is COPD?   1

Questions 1–15 define COPD and its causes, and provide fundamental information about the disorder, including:

- What is Chronic Obstructive Pulmonary Disorder?
- Is there a cure for COPD?

Part 2: COPD Complications and Associated Diseases   15

Questions 16–25 discuss and define respiratory failure, hyperinflated lungs, pneumonia, and other complications of COPD, including:

- Are there complications from COPD?
- Is depression a problem in patients with COPD?
- What is pulmonary bulla?

Part 3: Lung Function Monitoring   27

Questions 26–31 describe diagnostic tests and discuss their importance, including:

- Is early detection of COPD helpful?
- What are pulmonary function tests?
- What is spirometry?

Part 4: Living with COPD   35

Questions 32–53 cover exacerbation of COPD, the steps in a COPD action plan, and outline a checklist of medical tests and procedures, and other patient advice, including:

- I'm usually short of breath, even with minor exertion. How do I know if my COPD is getting worse?
- I don't want to bother my doctor unnecessarily about my illness. When should I call him about my symptoms?
- What is a "COPD action plan"?

This book was written with the patient and his or her family in mind. It provides useful information about chronic obstructive pulmonary disease (COPD) and helps the patient live a healthier and more comfortable life.

While the book can be read from cover to cover, it was designed as a reference text, so that a patient or caregiver can review particular questions and answers that are immediately important.

This book is not comprehensive in its scope and deals only with the most commonly asked questions. You can obtain additional information on resources and services for patients with COPD in the final chapter.

COPD Is Not a Death Sentence

"COPD is not a death sentence." These are the words of the late Bill Horden, COPD patient advocate and writer. And these are the words I clung to when diagnosed with severe COPD in August 2000.

That summer I began to have spells when I couldn't catch my breath while doing the simplest of activities. I was extremely short of breath most of the time and I was smoking way too many cigarettes.

Following a battery of tests, including a spirometry and arterial blood gas, my family doctor said, "It's bad, very, very bad." The words didn't scare me as much as the somber look on his face and the sad tone in his voice.

"You have severe emphysema," he said, "which is progressive and incurable." The next few minutes were a blur as he explained the diagnosis, interspersed with instructions for the nurse to order oxygen to be delivered to my home that very afternoon.

Oxygen! I thought. No, he can't be serious. Too stunned to ask questions, I nodded as he referred me to a pulmonary specialist and told me I needed to be in a pulmonary rehabilitation program.

That day my life changed forever. In a blink of an eye, I went from an independent, energetic newspaper editor with a bright future to a disabled chronically ill patient who had to rely on oxygen at night and medication by day to breathe more easily.

I tried to keep up with my fast-paced lifestyle, which now included three days a week at pulmonary rehab, but I couldn't. I simply did not have the energy. I took a leave of absence from work and fell into a deep depression.

I felt like I had become my illness. I had no life of my own—merely a life of survival—racing from doctor to doctor only to confirm what I already knew: at age 54, I had end-stage COPD caused by more than 30 years of smoking. I suffered in silence, wondering how long I had to live. Three years, five years? I didn't know and was too afraid to ask.

After months of living in limbo, I got downright angry and vowed I would not settle for a life that was defined by this illness. I turned to the Internet to learn all I could about COPD. The one thing I already knew was that pulmonary rehab was beginning to work miracles on my breathing and overall health.

While researching COPD online, I stumbled across the website of the late Bill Horden, known as the COPD Advocate. His positive words of wisdom gave me hope that I could not only live with COPD, but live well by becoming an informed patient and learning how to manage my disease.

I joined an online support group, where members shared their experiences of living with COPD. I learned that quitting smoking was the best thing I could do to slow the progression of my disease and that exercise was the key to keeping my energy levels up. I developed an attitude of gratitude, as many members were sicker than I was. When depressed, I spent time in the chat room with people who knew exactly how I was feeling.

Today my lifestyle does not revolve around my illness. I have adjusted to the fact that I have physical limitations and spend my precious energy wisely doing the things that are most important and meaningful to me. I am grateful for what I can do—even on days when I must slow down and rest because my breathing is more labored than usual.

My pulmonary function tests are almost the same as when I was first diagnosed four years ago. I attribute that gift to staying physically, mentally, and socially active and to staying connected to others who suffer from COPD.

In 2002, I retired from my full-time job with no regrets and followed my dream of living in a beach cottage on the eastern coast of the USA, where life is no longer a race to be endured, but a journey to be enjoyed—one breath at a time.

Susie Bowers

Susie Bowers is a retired journalist living in Rehoboth Beach, a town on the eastern coast of the United States. She is co-founder of www.copd-international.com, a nonprofit, interactive support site for people with chronic obstructive pulmonary disease and their caregivers.

She writes a weekly on-line newsletter and serves as website editor.

Reprinted with permission from Elsevier (Bowers. COPD Is Not a Death Sentence. Lancet 2004;364:896).

PART ONE

What is COPD?

What is Chronic Obstructive Pulmonary Disease?

Is there a cure for COPD?

More . . .

1. What is Chronic Obstructive Pulmonary Disease or COPD?

Chronic obstructive pulmonary disease (COPD)

several different lung diseases that share similar symptoms and demonstrate a similar pattern of dysfunction shown on spirometry.

Lungs

the primary respiratory organs in the chest; responsible for getting oxygen into the bloodstream and removing carbon dioxide.

Chronic obstructive pulmonary disease (COPD) is an umbrella term for diseases that restrict the flow of air out of the lungs.

Mucus

a clear, sticky mixture composed of water, proteins, and salts secreted by the mucus glands in the nose, sinuses, and airways of the lung.

COPD is a group of conditions that affect the lungs and airways. COPD stands for chronic (KRON-ick) obstructive (ob-STRUCK-tiv) pulmonary (PULL-muh-nair-ee) disease.

Chronic means that the condition is long term. You will have it the rest of your life. COPD usually gets worse over time, but you can learn how to manage it. *Pulmonary* refers to the **lungs** and airways. The condition is *obstructive* because it limits the flow of air into and out of your lungs. A *disease* is a disorder of body function, system, or organ.

Chronic obstructive pulmonary disease (COPD) is an umbrella term for diseases that restrict the flow of air out of the lungs. It is an all-inclusive, nonspecific term for chronic symptoms of cough, excess **mucus**, and exercise-related **dyspnea**. Emphysema and chronic **bronchitis** are the primary COPD diseases. COPD is a serious disorder of the lungs caused by chronic inflammation that results in the slow and progressive loss of lung function. The most common cause of COPD is smoking. The symptoms of COPD tend to get worse over time. While the most common and most characteristic symptom of COPD is shortness of breath, the symptoms of COPD can range from chronic cough and **sputum** production to severe disabling shortness of breath. **Hyperinflation** is a common symptom of COPD and can make it more difficult for the patient to breathe.

In some individuals, chronic cough and sputum production are the first signs that they are at risk for developing the air-flow obstruction and shortness of breath that are characteristic of COPD. In others, shortness of breath may be the first indication of the disease. COPD develops slowly, and it may be many years before the patient notices symptoms like shortness of breath. Most of the time, COPD is diagnosed in middle-aged or older people. Unlike people with asthma, the shortness of breath associated with COPD is only partially improved with medication.

Cecil's comment:

This is very true, and normal aging always worsens the symptoms. However, as a patient, I have found that there are ways to slow the progress of this illness and improve my quality of life: smoking cessation, exercise, education, diet, good medical support, and a positive mental attitude.

I have found that the concept of not being able to expel air rather than not getting enough air in is one of the hardest to understand. It is important to understand the concept and learn techniques to relieve this problem. It is beneficial that we know all about pursed-lip breathing and the proper lung exercises to help equalize the balance of oxygen and carbon dioxide in our system because they decrease the severity of anxiety attacks.

COPD is not just a disease of the lungs. Patients with COPD often lose a lot of body weight, including a significant loss of muscle mass, making COPD patients frail as well as short of breath. The amount of weight loss is related to how poorly the lungs work, with the sickest patients losing more than half their body weight. Not only is there a loss of muscle mass,

Dyspnea

shortness of breath, a subjective feeling of difficultly or distress in breathing.

Bronchitis

an inflammation of the bronchi, or small airways, in the lung, characterized by cough and sputum production.

Sputum

expectorated matter, especially mucus expectorated during diseases of the lung

Hyperinflation

a condition of the lungs in which the air sacs in the lungs lose their elasticity or stretchiness.

What is COPD?

but the remaining muscle does not function as well. This results in the patient's inability to work hard or exercise, which can reduce quality of life.

2. Does COPD have any other names?

Yes, chronic obstructive pulmonary disease is sometimes called chronic obstructive lung disease (COLD), emphysema, asthmatic bronchitis, and chronic bronchitis.

3. How are the lungs damaged in COPD?

The airways of the lung look like an upside-down tree, with branches becoming smaller and more numerous as you go downward and outward toward the edges of the lungs (Figure 1). At the end of each branch of the airway (called a **bronchiole**) are many small, balloon-like **air sacs** (called **alveoli**). In healthy people, each

Bronchiole

one of the smallest airways in the lung, near the alveoli.

Air sacs

also known as an alveolus, it is the space at the end of the smallest airway in the lung.

Alveoli

the small air sacs in the lung where oxygen is exchanged for carbon dioxide in the lung.

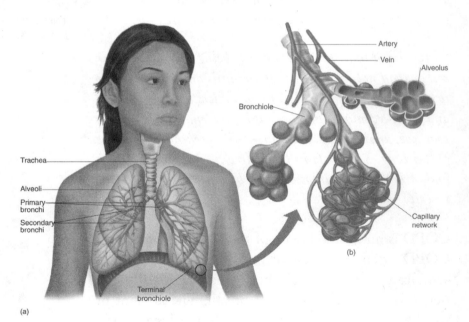

Figure 1   Lung anatomy

airway is clear and open; the air sacs are small and filled only with air. The branches and the air sacs are elastic and springy. When you breathe in, each air sac fills up with air, like a small balloon, and when you breathe out, the balloon deflates and the air goes out. In COPD, the airways and air sacs lose their shape and become floppy. The air has a harder time getting in and out of the branches and air sacs because they have lost their shape—they are blocked by mucus or are swollen shut. Sometimes, the walls between the air sacs are destroyed and there are fewer air sacs to supply oxygen to the blood.

4. Is COPD the same as emphysema and chronic bronchitis?

COPD is the term for a group of diseases that have many causes. Two of the main causes of COPD are emphysema and chronic bronchitis. Other diseases that can the cause COPD, although much less frequently, are asthma, **bronchiectasis**, **cystic fibrosis**, **pulmonary fibrosis**, and alpha-1 antitrypsin disease.

Doctors diagnose **chronic bronchitis** in patients who have daily cough and sputum production that lasts at least 3 months for at least 2 consecutive years. While chronic bronchitis can lead to COPD, not all people with chronic bronchitis progress to severe shortness of breath. Certain changes occur in the lungs of people with chronic bronchitis. Specifically, the airways become inflamed and thickened, and there is an increase in the number and size of the cells that produce mucus. This results in excessive mucus production, leading to cough and difficulty getting air in and

Bronchiectasis
a chronic dilation of the airways in the lung as the result of chronic inflammation. This condition is often associated with infections and increased sputum production.

Cystic fibrosis
a genetic disorder that affects the lungs. The lining of the lungs produces excess mucus. This mucus clogs the small breathing passages, making it difficult to breathe.

Pulmonary fibrosis
a disease of the lungs in which normal lung tissue is replaced with fibroctic (or scar) tissue. When the scar forms, the lung tissue becomes thicker and less able to transfer oxygen into the bloodstream. This process is irreversible.

Chronic bronchitis
a chronic disease characterized by coughing and sputum production that last for at least 3 months in 2 consecutive years.

What is COPD?

out of the lungs. The chronic inflammation and excessive mucus production cause lung damage and shortness of breath.

Emphysema
a disease of the lungs that causes severe shortness of breath.

The shortness of breath in **emphysema** comes through a different mechanism. In emphysema, the walls of the air sacs (or alveoli) in the lungs are destroyed, leading to the formation of a few large air sacs, instead of many tiny ones. The lung begins to look like a sponge with many large bubbles or holes in it, instead of a sponge with very even tiny holes. These few large air sacs do not work as well as the many tiny air sacs and are less able to supply the blood with oxygen. When the blood cannot get enough oxygen, the patient becomes short of breath. Cough is not common in the early part of the emphysema type of COPD, but it can occur late in the disease. Most people with COPD have a combination of both chronic bronchitis and emphysema.

Cecil's comment:

The older terminology for these two types of COPD is "pink puffers" and "blue bloaters." The pink puffers are usually patients with low weight who have very little cough and have a pinkish tint to their skin. The predominant component of their COPD is emphysema. The blue bloater is different, in that their major component of COPD is bronchitis, and they sometimes have a light gray or bluish tint to their lips and fingernails. They are usually bloated, overweight, and susceptible to mucus build-up and a cough.

5. Is COPD the same as asthma?

COPD has a lot in common with asthma. Both diseases tend to run in families; both are caused by inflammation that causes narrowing of the airways (called bronchospasm); both have reversible components or both can be progressive. Sometimes, it is difficult to separate asthma from COPD, and, indeed, the diseases may coexist. However, the cause of COPD is quite different from that of asthma, and the course of the two diseases is always very different.

Although the term asthma is sometimes used interchangeably with COPD to describe patients with chronic shortness of breath, they are not exactly the same. **Asthma** is a common disease of the lungs and is often first diagnosed in children. Although asthma can be worsened by smoking, it is not caused by smoking. Like COPD, asthma is characterized by shortness of breath, but medication tends to completely reverse the airway blockage; in COPD, the blockage is not completely reversible. Asthma does not necessarily follow a course of worsening shortness of breath as COPD does. Some scientists believe that in a small percentage of cases, asthma can lead to COPD.

Cecil's comment:

I have known several people whose COPD was misdiagnosed. This occasionally happens because the symptoms of COPD and advanced asthma are similar.

6. What is the prognosis of patients with COPD?

The overall prognosis of a patient with COPD depends on the severity of the patient's lung disease at diagnosis and whether the patient continues to smoke. The severity of the lung disease can be estimated by doctors by using a lung measurement test called spirometry. One of the measures of lung function is the

---

Bronchospasm

a contraction of the smooth muscle in the airways that results in narrower air passages and difficulty breathing.

Asthma

an inflammatory disease of the lung that results in reversible airway obstruction. Unlike COPD, asthma's symptoms tend to wax and wane in severity.

The overall prognosis of a patient with COPD depends on the severity of the patient's lung disease at diagnosis and whether the patient continues to smoke.

What is COPD?

7

Forced expiratory volume after 1 second (FEV1)

a common spirometric measurement of the volume of air that can be breathed out in 1 second.

forced expiratory volume after 1 second (FEV1). The FEV1 is a measure of the maximum amount of air that person can breath out in one second. If a patient with COPD has an FEV1 that is at least 50% of what a normal person the same height and age can breathe out, then he or she has a very good prognosis, with the survival of these patients being only slightly less than that of patients without COPD. Patients with an FEV1 of less than 0.75 L (very severe obstruction, less than 30% of that predicted) have a 1-year mortality rate of 30% and a 10-year mortality rate of 95%. No matter how poor a COPD patient's lung impairment is, the patient's prognosis improves if he or she quits smoking.

7. Who gets COPD?

The vast majority of patients, approximately 90%, who are diagnosed with COPD are or were heavy cigarette smokers for many years. Not all smokers get COPD. Fifty percent of patients who smoke have measurable lung damage, and in approximately 20% of patients, this develops into COPD. There is also a relationship between the amount of cigarettes smoked and the risk of developing COPD. The greater the number of packs per day, the greater the number of years of smoking, the greater the risk of COPD.

Breathing in other kinds of lung irritants, like pollution, dust, or chemicals over a long period of time, may also cause or contribute to COPD, although this is much less common. This type of COPD may occur in firefighters, farmers, bakers, or workers in chemical plants. COPD occurs predominantly in individuals older than 40 years. Although COPD is still much more common in men than in women, the greatest increase in the COPD death rate between 1979 and 1989 occurred in women, particularly in black women (117.6 percent for black women vs. 93 percent for white women).

8. Why is the rate of COPD increasing in women?

These increases in COPD among women probably reflect the increase in smoking by women since the 1940s. In the United States, a history of currently or formerly smoking is the risk factor most often linked to COPD, and the increase in the number of women smoking over the past half century is mirrored in the increase in COPD rates among women.

9. What causes COPD?

While COPD can have many causes, the most common cause is lung tissue destruction from inhaled irritants. The lungs and airways are highly sensitive to inhaled irritants. Prolonged exposure to inhaled irritants can lead to inflamed and narrowed air passages that make it difficult to inhale and exhale. The elastic fibers in the lung that allow the lung to stretch, then come back to its resting shape, are damaged. This makes breathing air in and out of the lungs more difficult.

Cigarette smoking is the most common irritant that causes COPD. Pipe, cigar, and other types of tobacco smoking can also cause COPD, especially if the smoke is inhaled. Other causes of COPD can be genetic, such as cystic fibrosis or alpha-1 antitrypsin disease, although this is rare. In the third world, indoor pollution is a significant cause of COPD, particularly the smoke from heating and cooking fires.

10. Aside from tobacco smoke, can other toxins or pollutants cause COPD?

Smoking is the main cause of COPD, but other causes should not be overlooked. In a new study of 2000 adults with COPD in the United States, researchers from the University of California found that exposure to airborne toxins at work may cause one in five cases of chronic lung disease. The disease is actually twice as common among those who are exposed to toxins during the course of their job, such as miners, metalworkers, bakers, firefighters, or farmers. Those who also smoked were even more at risk. A smoker who was exposed to toxins at work had 18 times the risk of COPD of a nonsmoker who was not exposed to occupational toxins. This study suggests that employers should do more to reduce exposure to health hazards at work.

As we can clearly see, patients with COPD who breathe fumes and dusts may worsen their disease. Some examples of lung irritants that patients should avoid include

- Working around certain kinds of chemicals and breathing in the fumes for many years (e.g., chemical factory workers, firefighters)
- Working in a dusty area over many years (e.g., coal miners, farmers)
- Heavy exposure to air pollution. (e.g., toll booth workers, car mechanics)
- Being around second-hand smoke, which is smoke in the air from other people smoking cigarettes (e.g., spouses of smokers, waitresses, and bartenders)

Cecil's comment:

Excess mold and mildew can be a lung irritant. If your home has large amounts of mold or mildew, this problem should be investigated. You can normally get information on testing your home at your local Health Department, or you can contact your Environmental Protection Agency (EPA) representative in your area.

11. I've heard that the rate of COPD in the United States is decreasing. Is that true?

Yes, the overall rate of mild-to-moderate COPD is decreasing in the United States (although the rate of COPD is increasing worldwide). The decreases in rates of mild and moderate COPD in both men and women aged 25–54 years in the past quarter century reflect the decrease in overall smoking rates in the United States since the 1960s. However, the rates in certain groups in the United States is increasing, such as in women and minorities. This reflects an increase in the rates of smoking in these groups.

12. Is COPD serious?

Yes, COPD is a very serious disease in the United States. More than 13.5 million Americans are thought to have COPD, and it is the fifth leading cause of death in the United States. Between 1980 and 1990, the total death rate from COPD increased by 22%. In 1990, it was estimated that 84,000 deaths resulted from COPD, approximately 34 per 100,000 people. Within the next 15 years, it is estimated that COPD will become the third most common form of death worldwide. It is a growing public health issue. Furthermore, COPD decreases the overall quality of life of patients by robbing them of physical vitality and the ability to socialize and work.

13. Is there a cure for COPD?

No, there is no cure for COPD. The damage to a patient's airways and lungs cannot be reversed. The encouraging news is that in most cases you can halt, or at least greatly slow, the progression of emphysema if you quit smoking. There are things that you can do to feel better and slow the damage to the lungs, such as avoiding lung irritants and infections, taking medication as prescribed, and getting involved in a rehabilitation program.

Cecil's comment:

Although there is no known cure for COPD, it is important that each patient realize that this is not a death sentence but a change in lifestyle. Living with this illness is easier if you take control of your life and work with your physician to manage the symptoms of the disease. Another point to remember is that you should have hope. Major strides have been made in the past decade in the research and development of medications and procedures to improve and lengthen the life span of patients with COPD.

14. Can COPD be prevented, and is it contagious?

Yes, COPD can be prevented. Avoiding cigarette smoking and second-hand smoke is most important way to prevent COPD. Other prevention strategies include avoiding environments or work sites that contain lung irritants and air pollutants, such as dust, fumes, and chemicals. If you must work in such an environment, wearing appropriate safety masks and ventilators when working with lung irritants is also recommended. Avoiding respiratory infections and

The encouraging news is that in most cases you can halt, or at least greatly slow, the progression of emphysema if you quit smoking. There are things that you can do to feel better and slow the damage to the lungs, such as avoiding lung irritants and infections, taking medication as prescribed, and getting involved in a rehabilitation program.

getting appropriate influenza and pneumococcal **vaccines** is also helpful in preventing COPD because chronic lung infections can worsen the condition of patients with decreased lung function.

COPD is not a contagious disease. One cannot catch it from someone else

15. I read in the newspaper that COPD is often undetected and untreated. Is that true?

Well, yes and no. COPD is detected by people who suffer from it. Their symptoms are obvious to them, but the symptoms come on slowly for the most part, and people accommodate to less activity over years. This is especially true of smokers, who tend to cough more and bring up more **phlegm** and feel that shortness of breath is just part of smoking, so they tend not to report it to their doctor. Also, because most patients are 45 years of age or older, many think shortness of breath is a common part of the aging process. You might say that the symptoms of COPD are always detected but not recognized as being part of a disease.

On the other hand, if doctors were more aggressive about asking patients about these symptoms and testing those at risk, more people would be diagnosed. This is especially alarming in light of studies that have estimated that 70% of smokers see a primary care clinician at least once each year for some reason. Regular review of the smoking and brief symptom history, as well as use of the simple office spirometer, can identify patients

Vaccine

a specialized preparation designed to stimulate the body's system to make protective antibodies directed against specific bacteria or viruses.

What is COPD?

Phlegm

abnormal amounts of mucus, especially as expectorated from the mouth. Often a sign of inflammation or infection.

who could be saved from late symptomatic stages of COPD by smoking cessation and other interventions.

These two facets of the same problem explain the results of a study conducted by the US Centers for Disease Control and Prevention (CDC), which found that at least two thirds of people with lung disease are not aware that they have it.

Cecil's comment:

Through working with patient support groups, I have found that many patients do not know or understand the full effect of the disease until they have a major exacerbation and are admitted into the hospital, and usually put in the intensive care unit (ICU) on a ventilator. I have known patients who go into the hospital with an unknown diagnosis and are released on oxygen 24/7 and are seriously disabled. It is extremely important that the diagnosis is accompanied by proper counseling for patients. In my experience, too many leave the hospital after hearing "COPD" and write to support groups like us to find out just what it means and how to manage it. COPD is not just a disease of the lungs.

There are so many minor and major complications or ailments that are more likely to occur with this illness. Too many patients have a tendency to blame problems on aging and live with them on a daily basis. Any time you have any symptom that affects how you feel or decreases your ability to accomplish your daily routine, you should consult with your physician, who can tell you whether it is the result of normal aging or COPD.

PART TWO

COPD
Complications and Associated Diseases

Are there complications from COPD?

Is depression a problem in patients with COPD?

What is a pulmonary bulla?

More ...

16. Are there complications from COPD?

Yes, COPD is a serious disease, and it has complications that involve the lung and other organs in your body. These complications include

- Cor pulmonale (a type of heart failure)
- Lower leg swelling (edema)
- Acute COPD exacerbations (sudden, serious worsening of your shortness of breath)
- Respiratory distress
- Respiratory failure
- Hyperinflated lungs
- Polycythemia (thickening of the blood)
- Pulmonary bullae
- Pneumothorax (a rupture of the lung)
- Pneumonia
- Bronchiectasis
- Depression
- Loss of body weight and muscle mass
- Gastroesophageal reflux disease (GERD)

These complications are described more fully below.

Cor Pulmonale

Cor pulmonale is a complication of COPD that results in high blood pressure in the lungs and poor functioning of the muscles in the right side of the heart. COPD makes the heart work harder, especially the right side, which pumps blood into the lungs. COPD causes low levels of oxygen in the blood, causing blood vessels to constrict. Many of the capillaries, the very small blood vessels that surround the alveoli, are destroyed in the disease process. This makes the

Cor pulmonale

acute strain or hypertrophy of the right ventricle caused by a disorder of the lungs or of the pulmonary blood vessels.

heart work harder because it has to force blood through fewer constricted blood vessels. As a result of this effort, the right ventricle becomes enlarged, the walls of the heart thicken, and the chamber eventually loses its ability to contract efficiently.

Respiratory Distress

Respiratory distress is a condition in which there is not enough oxygen in the blood because the lungs are less able to take in oxygen. When you are in respiratory distress, you may be short of breath and you may get out of breath by doing simple tasks, such as walking across a room or brushing your teeth. Respiratory distress can lead to respiratory failure.

Respiratory distress
difficulty breathing, visibly labored breathing.

Respiratory Failure

Respiratory failure is a life-threatening situation in which the respiratory system stops functioning properly. Respiratory failure occurs when the lungs and respiratory system are unable to provide the body with sufficient oxygen and fail to "blow off" accumulated carbon dioxide. "Hypoxemic" respiratory failure is the inability of the lungs to take in enough oxygen to meet the body's oxygen requirement. "Hypercapnic" respiratory failure occurs when carbon dioxide levels rise within the body because the lungs are unable to get rid of it fast enough. It is not unusual for a patient to have both situations at the same time (called a "mixed pattern" of respiratory failure).

Respiratory failure
the inability of your lungs to keep up.

Respiratory failure can be very gradual and may progress slowly over months to years. This is called "chronic respiratory failure." Most patients with

COPD have chronic respiratory failure. Acute respiratory failure is characterized by a sudden onset of shortness of breath that occurs over hours or days. This can occur in patients with COPD when they acquire a lung infection or are exposed to lung irritants that cause inflammation and increased mucus production.

In both acute and chronic respiratory failure, there can come a point where the failure becomes so marked that the body becomes deprived of oxygen or the level of carbon dioxide is too high (severe respiratory failure). When these conditions occur, other organs can begin to fail as well from the lack of oxygen. The brain is particularly sensitive to lack of oxygen and build-up of carbon dioxide. In this state, the patient can become confused, unable to make appropriate decisions about his or her own treatment, possibly lose consciousness, and go into a coma. If this state is prolonged, the oxygen levels become too low, and the patient can die. Clearly, severe respiratory failure is a medical emergency; the patient is critically ill and requires the attention of a physician and sometimes needs to be admitted to the hospital. Because of the effect of respiratory failure on the brain, it is inappropriate to allow the patient in severe failure to make decisions about visiting the doctor or emergency room. In this situation, a relative or friend must make decisions for the patient and get him or her the proper emergency care.

Hyperinflated Lungs

You have about 300 million air sacs (alveoli) in each lung. The walls of these air sacs contain elastic fibers that allow them to expand and contract like small balloons when you breathe. When these walls are damaged, as they are in COPD, they lose their elasticity. Because they are unable to contract properly, more air remains in the air sacs when you exhale and overstretches (hyperinflates) them. The hyperinflated air sacs cannot force air out of your lungs as well as the small air sacs when you exhale. For this reason, you have to breathe harder just to get enough oxygen in your blood.

Pneumonia

Pneumonia is common in COPD because the lungs are less able to clear bacteria out of the airways. It is caused by bacterial infection that can lead to respiratory failure in patients with COPD. *Streptococcus pneumoniae* is the most common cause of bacterial pneumonia in patients with COPD.

Cecil's comment:

Pneumonia is area of grave concern for us as patients. It is fairly common for a COPD patient to become a little more short of breath and feel worse than usual. Some just accept this as a bad breathing day. Any changes in breathing should be reported to your doctor or an emergency plan should be put into action if you have already discussed this issue with your doctor. In reality, it can be pneumonia and we would not realize it.

Pneumothorax

Pneumothorax occurs when a hole develops in the lung, allowing air to escape into the space between the lung and the chest wall and collapsing the lung. Patients with COPD are at increased risk for spontaneously developing these holes because of their weakened lung structure. A pneumothorax can lead to severe respiratory distress and is treated by inserting a tube into the space between the lung and the chest wall (pleural space) to allow the air to escape out of the

Pneumonia

an infection of one or both lungs that is usually caused by a bacterium, virus, or fungus. Patients with COPD are at increased risk for pneumonia.

Pneumonia is common in COPD because the lungs are less able to clear bacteria out of the airways.

Pneumothorax

a condition in which air gets between your lungs and your chest wall.

space and then re-expanding the lung. The tube must remain in the space until the hole is repaired.

Polycythemia

Polycythemia in COPD is the body's attempt to adjust to decreased amounts of blood oxygen by increasing the production of oxygen-carrying red blood cells. While this may be helpful in the short term, overproduction of red blood cells eventually clogs small blood vessels.

Polycythemia

an increase above normal in the number of red cells in the blood.

Gastroesophageal Reflux Disease

Gastroesophageal reflux disease (GERD) is also known as acid reflux disease. This condition is increasingly common among persons with progressive COPD. More than half of those with advanced COPD have GERD. This is important because acid reflux can cause pain that mimics heart disease, which may confuse the patient and the physician and require expensive testing to tell the difference. Also, acid reflux is associated, in some cases, with worsening of COPD symptoms, which occurs when acid reflux is inhaled into the lungs, causing inflammation, wheezing, and shortness of breath. It is also important to remember that several commonly used COPD medications, including beta agonists, theophylline, and corticosteroids, can exacerbate GERD.

Gastroesophageal reflux disease (GERD)

a condition that occurs when acid in the stomach enters the esophagus. It is the cause of "heart burn" or "agita."

17. Is depression a problem in COPD?

Yes. Depression occurs frequently in the general population and even more frequently in patients with diseases like COPD. The worsening of symptoms of COPD has a detrimental effect on the patient's lifestyle and ability to cope with daily living. There-

Depression occurs frequently in the general population and even more frequently in patients with diseases like COPD.

fore, it is frequently associated with depression or anxiety; in fact, depression occurs in more than 20% of patients diagnosed with COPD.

Because depression is a disorder that is easily missed by physicians because of its nonspecific symptoms, it should be brought to their attention by either the patient or his or her family or friends. Common symptoms of depression that should be looked out for include

- Changes in appetite
- Sudden loss or gain in weight
- Changes in sleep patterns (either sleeplessness or waking too early)
- Feelings of guilt, hopelessness, and despair
- Mental and physical fatigue
- Inability to make decisions
- Withdrawal from others
- Lack of pleasure in once-pleasurable activities
- Thoughts of death and suicide

If depression is identified, it can be treated and the quality of the patient's life improved. Treatment for depressed COPD patients is the same as that for patients without COPD. Treatment strategies include counseling, education, frequent patient monitoring, and medications. These have a high success rate.

Cecil's comment:

Depression is commonly associated with COPD. It can be one of the most devastating side effects of our illness. If you let depression get a foothold, then it will affect your ability to function properly and will rob you of the initiative to fight this illness and "stay on top" of everything that is going on in your life. Your mind is your most important asset in handling all the physical aspects of your disease. Do not feel that depression is a sign of mental weakness or that it is something to be ashamed of. Depression can be effectively treated with medication. If the first medication doesn't help, then continue to work with your doctor until you find one that does. Don't give up on the first few tries.

Dr. Quinn mentions that guilt is a common symptom of depression. I agree and have noticed that there is a tendency for patients with COPD to assume the blame for their illness as a result of their history of smoking. Self blame only worsens depression and anxiety. It is a good idea to absolve yourself of blame and move on. Assuming guilt for our disease only hinders our treatment—focusing on medical treatments and self care is much more productive.

18. Is bronchiectasis part of COPD?

Bronchiectasis

a chronic dilation of the airways in the lung as the result of chronic inflammation.

Yes, **bronchiectasis** can be a complication of COPD as well as a rare cause of COPD. It begins as an abnormal stretching and enlarging of the respiratory passages, caused by mucus blockage. When the mucus cannot be cleared from the airways in the lung, it becomes stuck and accumulates in those airways. The blockage causes inflammation, which further blocks the airway and decreases the chance that the mucus blockage can be cleared. Bacterial infections can develop in these blocked areas, leading to further inflammation and scarring. A cycle of blockage, inflammation, and infection leaves the air passages scarred and deformed. This is often misdiagnosed as recurrent pneumonia or even asthma.

19. Are the symptoms of bronchiectasis different from those of emphysema–type COPD?

Not really. The symptoms of bronchiectasis are similar to those of other COPD types and include coughing, fever, weakness, weight loss, and fatigue. Coughing occurs more frequently when the patient is lying down because mucus accumulates and may be associated with chest pain in the area of the blockage and infection. Patients with bronchiectasis may cough up thick, foul-smelling sputum.

20. How can the doctor detect bronchiectasis?

The doctor can detect bronchiectasis by eliciting a history of frequent episodes of shortness of breath, fever, and cough productive of thick, foul-smelling sputum. The doctor can order a chest x-ray study, breathing tests (spirometry), sputum culture, bronchoscopy, or computed tomography (CT) scan, which are helpful in making the diagnosis. Some diseases occur commonly with bronchiectasis, such as cystic fibrosis and tuberculosis. The doctor may check for them if he or she suspects bronchiectasis. If the cycle of blockages, infection, and scarring is broken early, the air passages may return to normal function. Therefore, early treatment with antibiotics and bronchodilators is important. Similarly, avoiding infections by getting vaccinations against influenza, measles, and pneumococcus infection is recommended. Finally, as with all patients with COPD, bronchiectasis patients should avoid cigarette smoke and other irritants that may inflame the lungs.

21. How is bronchiectasis treated?

Patients with bronchiectasis are often given antibiotics for infection and bronchodilator medicines to open air passages. Physical therapy techniques may be used to help clear mucus. Lobectomies and lung transplantations are also an option for severe cases.

22. What is a pulmonary bulla?

Bulla (bullae)

large, thin-walled air sacs in the lung, composed of the remains of many disrupted and distended smaller air sacs.

A **bulla** is a bubble-like structure found on the edges of the lung. It is an air-filled space larger than 1 centimeter, but it can grow over months to years into a large air sac. These enlarged bullae can cause symptoms by compression of normal lung tissue. Additionally, bullae can fill with fluid and become infected, or they can rupture and leak air between the lung and the chest wall (pneumothorax.) A pneumothorax is a medical emergency that requires surgery (Figure 2).

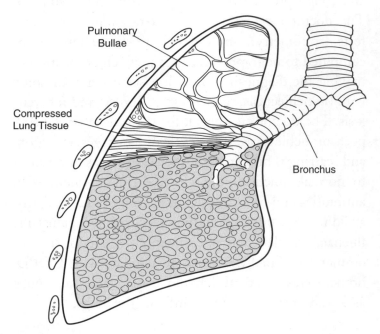

Figure 2   Pulmonary Bullae

23. What is bullous emphysema?

Bullous emphysema is emphysema that is complicated with enlarged airspaces (bullae) around the edges of the lung. These bullae usually measure 1 to several centimeters in diameter, and they are often visible on chest x-ray studies or CT scans. They can occur as a solitary bulla or as many bullae. These thin-walled air sacs are inflated with inhaled air and have a higher air pressure than the surrounding lung tissue. They can compress nearby healthy lung tissue and keep it from functioning properly.

24. How is bullous emphysema treated?

The shortness of breath, caused by the compression of normal lung tissue by the inflated bullae, can be improved with surgical removal of the bullae.

25. I have a friend with alpha-1 antitrypsin deficiency. Is that the same as COPD?

Although alpha-1 antitrypsin (AAT) deficiency is a well-established cause of COPD, it is not a common cause of COPD. In fact, AAT deficiency accounts for only 1% of all cases of COPD. AAT deficiency results from a genetic defect, which results in the lack of production of a liver protein that blocks the destructive effects of certain enzymes. The condition may lead to emphysema and liver disease. Approximately 75% of adults with severe deficiency of AAT will develop emphysema, which often begins before 40 years of age. Individuals who have AAT who also smoke have a greatly increased risk of developing a severe form of COPD called panlobular emphysema before the age of 35.

COPD Complications and Associated Diseases

Cecil's comment:

While working with a large support group, I have found that very few people are ever informed of the possibility of alpha-1 antitrypsin disease. If you have family members with COPD, especially if they have never smoked, then you should consult with your doctor about taking the test for AAT deficiency. It is simply a blood test that can be administered in a few minutes, but it can make a big difference if you are found to have AAT deficiency because the treatments for it are somewhat different than that for other forms of COPD.

PART THREE

Lung Function Monitoring

Is early detection of COPD helpful?

What are pulmonary function tests?

What is spirometry?

More . . .

26. Is early detection of COPD helpful?

Yes, even if the patient has a long history of smoking or exposure to other lung irritants, early detection and treatment of COPD can slow down or stop the damage to your lungs. The stage of the disease can suggest the prognosis of the disease. Although moderate and severe cases of COPD are associated with a higher death rate, those who are diagnosed with milder disease can enjoy a normal life span if their disease does not progress. The doctor can detect COPD by examination and spirometry in these people, many of whom have no respiratory symptoms. The earlier that you are diagnosed, the earlier you can be treated and the healthier you will be.

Even if the patient has a long history of smoking or exposure to other lung irritants, early detection and treatment of COPD can slow down or stop the damage to your lungs.

The key to the diagnosis of all stages of COPD is simple spirometric measurements, which can and should be used regularly in all patients who are at risk. Your doctor can perform the simple, painless test called spirometry to measure your pulmonary function and detect COPD. Spirometry is recommended for patients who are current smokers or who were smokers in the past, those smokers aged 45 years and older, as well as anyone with persistent respiratory problems, such as chronic cough, chronic sputum production, or shortness of breath during mild exercise.

Cecil's comment:

I have found that in most cases, early diagnosis has allowed the patient to take the proper precautions to stop, or in a few cases, slightly reverse the symptoms in this disease. The earlier the diagnosis, the better chance of living a longer, healthier, more productive life.

27. What diagnostic tests are most helpful in diagnosing COPD?

The most helpful diagnostic tests used in diagnosing COPD are pulmonary function tests (PFTs). Other useful tests are blood tests and x-ray studies.

Blood tests are useful for getting an overall picture of a person's health, as well as excluding other diagnoses. For example, alpha-1 antitrypsin disease can be diagnosed with a blood test.

Most doctors order a chest x-ray study for people suspected of having COPD. A chest x-ray study provides a picture of the heart and lungs and is routinely used to help evaluate shortness of breath, a major symptom of COPD. It can also help support a diagnosis of COPD. Plain x-ray studies and CT scans of the chest allow doctors to see the heart, lungs, and surrounding tissues. These tests can identify bullae, tumors, pneumonias, a collapsed lung, an enlarged heart, and abnormal fluid collections in the chest, which are common diagnoses for people with shortness of breath. A normal x-ray study does not mean that a person does not have COPD; in fact, in milder cases of COPD, the lungs may appear normal on chest x-ray study or CT scan. However, in severe cases of COPD, the x-ray findings are common and may include

- Flattening of the diaphragm
- Increased size of the chest, as measured from front to back
- A long, narrow heart
- Hyperinflation (when COPD is severe, and air is trapped in the lungs, the lungs appear larger than nor-

mal on a chest x-ray study; doctors call this "hyper-inflation," which is a classic x-ray sign of COPD)

- Abnormal air collections within the lung (focal bullae)

Although a chest x-ray study can detect advanced emphysema, this test alone cannot otherwise diagnose COPD. A chest x-ray study should always be performed at the time of initial diagnosis of COPD. Although routine scheduled follow-up chest x-ray studies are not recommended, many doctors advise smokers and recent ex-smokers to have this test every 1–2 years.

28. What are pulmonary function tests?

Pulmonary function tests (PFTs) are designed to measure lung function. Although they were originally created as tools for researchers who studied the lungs, they are now widely available and commonly used in both specialist and generalist offices to detect lung disease.

The term PFTs is used to describe a group of lung tests. The first and most common is spirometry.

Cecil's comment:

This is an area where patient involvement is critical. If your doctor schedules you for a PFT and you are not feeling well, have an infection, or have other environmental factors that are affecting your breathing, then you should notify your doctor and have the test rescheduled until you are in your best condition. This test is an indicator to your doctor of many important things. It provides an indication of how stable your lungs are, as well as valuable information about how your medications are working and whether medication changes or adjustments are required. Most importantly, these results

---

Pulmonary function tests (PFTs) are designed to measure lung function. Although they were originally created as tools for researchers who studied the lungs, they are now widely available and commonly used in both specialist and generalist offices to detect lung disease.

Pulmonary function tests (PFTs)

tests of lung function that include measurements of lung volumes, breathing capacity, and gas diffusion.

are reviewed when any type of operation or procedure is required. Flawed results could affect the decision on whether to proceed.

29. What is spirometry?

Spirometry is the most commonly performed test of lung function, and it is the most reliable way to diagnose many obstructive lung diseases, like asthma and COPD. It is performed using a machine called a spirometer. Spirometry is a quick, noninvasive, and painless way to see whether there is damage to your lung and to diagnose COPD.

The spirometer is a machine that measures how much air you breathe out and in, and how quickly you can do it. The patient inhales as deeply as possible and forms a seal around the tube with the mouth. Then the patient exhales, as forcefully and rapidly as possible, until the patient can exhale no more. For the test to be adequate, the patient must exhale all the air he or she possibly can continue exhaling for at least another 6 seconds. Usually, three separate attempts are made, and the best result is used for evaluation. The spirometer then calculates the amount of air the lungs can hold and the rate that air can be inhaled and exhaled. The spirometry measurements are printed out in both a graph format and a numerical format. The results of the test are compared with those of healthy individuals of similar height and age, and of the same sex and race.

Spirometry gives the doctor two important readings: the peak expiratory flow (PEF) and the FEV1. The PEF and FEV1 values reflect your ability to empty your lungs efficiently.

Spirometry

a method of making lung function measurements using a device called a spirometer.

The FEV1 is a common spirometry measurement of the volume of air that can be breathed out in 1 second. For patients with COPD, FEV1 is used to determine the severity of the obstruction. For example, if your FEV1 is less than 70%, your COPD is considered mild. If it is less than 35%, your COPD is considered severe.

Cecil's comment:

The FEV1 is a very important number for us COPD patients. It is used by the doctor to track the progression of the illness. It is also used by physicians when managing your medications.

The PEF is the maximum flow of air that can be exhaled in the beginning of a forced **expiration**.

Expiration

the act of breathing out, or exhaling.

When a person has severe COPD, air gets trapped in the air sacs of the lungs, and the airways get swollen and clogged with phlegm. When this person exhales, not all the air leaves the lungs because of the air trapping, and so the amount of air leaving the lungs is lower than that of a normal person of the same age and height, leading to a lower FEV1 value. Similarly, if the patient has to exhale through constricted and phlegm-clogged airways, the flow of air is decreased, affecting the PEF, which measures the maximum flow of air during a forced exhalation.

Total lung volume

the amount of air that is contained in the lungs after a deep inspiration.

Forced vital capacity (FVC)

the maximum volume of gas that can be forcefully and rapidly expired after a maximal inspiration.

Spirometry also measures the total amount of air that your lung holds (**total lung volume**), as well as the total amount of air that you can breathe in and out (**forced vital capacity**). As COPD gets more severe, the amount of air in your lungs (total lung volume) may increase, through air trapping, but the amount of air that you can breathe in and out (your vital capacity) may decrease.

Cecil's comment:

When spirometry is used to diagnose COPD, a patient should make sure that follow-up tests are performed to confirm the diagnosis. As Dr. Quinn stated, the testing for the presence and the progression of the disease should be accomplished with an ABG test, an x-ray study of the chest, and a full set of PFTs. Do not assume that spirometry alone can diagnose the disease.

30. Why should I have spirometry?

Spirometry is a fast, painless, and accurate way to measure lung function and diagnose COPD. If you have a history of smoking, or if the doctor suspects from your medical history and physical examination that you have lung disease, spirometry will help confirm this diagnosis. If you are diagnosed and treated early, you can have improved health and less disability from COPD.

31. What is a gas diffusion test?

A **gas diffusion test** measures how well oxygen and other gases pass through the lung's air sacs and are absorbed by the blood. During this test, you are asked to breath in a small amount of gas called carbon monoxide. This gas diffuses through the lung tissue and is absorbed by the blood. The gas then can be measured in your blood, and the result is called your gas **diffusion capacity**. Like other lung function tests, the amount of gas that is absorbed by your lungs is compared with that of people with normal lung function. If your gas diffusion capacity is low, your lungs

Gas diffusion test
used to determine how well oxygen and other gases pass from the air sacs of the lungs into the blood.

Diffusion capacity
a test used to determine how well oxygen passes from the air sacs of the lungs into the blood; also known as lung diffusion testing.

33

are not absorbing gases as well as they should, and it could indicate that you have COPD.

Cecil's comment:

If you are claustrophobic or have reservations about close spaces, then it would be wise to discuss this portion of the test with your doctor or the respiratory therapist. The chamber is similar to a phone booth and is completely sealed.

The American Lung Association encourages spirometry for everyone who is a smoker older than 45 years or anyone who regularly experiences breathlessness, has difficulty breathing, or otherwise suspects that he or she has a lung disease.

PART FOUR

Living with COPD

I'm usually short of breath, even with minor exertion. How do I know if my COPD is getting worse?

I don't want to bother my doctor unnecessarily about my illness. When should I call him about my symptoms? What is a "COPD action plan"?

More . . .

32. I'm usually short of breath, even with minor exertion. How do I know if my COPD is getting worse?

Because early treatment of worsening COPD is most effective in preventing hospitalizations, it is very important for the patient to recognize when symptoms are getting worse. The early symptoms or warning signs of a COPD exacerbation can be different for each person. You are the best person to know whether you are having difficulty breathing, but family members or friends may also recognize some of these signs. Therefore, it is important that you inform your family and friends of these warning signs. A change or increase in the symptoms you usually experience may be the only early warning sign. You may notice one or more of the following:

- Any change in sputum, including the amount, color, odor, and thickness/stickiness, or if you notice any blood in the sputum
- Any worsening of your shortness of breath, cough, or wheezing, especially if it is associated with fever or interferes with your usual daily activities or your ability to sleep
- Waking up more than once per night with shortness of breath
- Ankle, lower leg, or hand swelling
- Prolonged headache, forgetfulness, confusion, slurring of speech, and sleepiness
- Use of more pillows or sleeping in a chair instead of a bed to avoid shortness of breath
- An unexplained increase or decrease in weight
- Any feeling of ill health, increased fatigue, and lack of energy that continues for more than 24 hours

- Any blue color in your lips or fingernails

All patients with COPD should have an **action plan** to deal with worsening symptoms. The action plan should be developed with the help of your doctor and discussed with your family, friends, or caregivers.

Cecil's comments:

If you live alone and you have an exacerbation, regardless of the severity, you should have someone contact you at least two to three times a day. This person can also assist with your daily chores, such as shopping and cooking. Never be so independent that you do not ask for help when it is needed. You are not being a burden on your friends and loved ones. If you have no other resources, you may contact your church or ask your doctor about visiting nurse services or volunteer services for these purposes.

33. I don't want to bother my doctor unnecessarily about my illness. When should I call him about my symptoms?

If severe symptoms are present, it is vital to begin the appropriate treatment immediately. Symptoms do not go away when they are ignored. Therefore, knowing when to call your health care provider is very important in managing your chronic lung disease. Working with your doctor is very important in determining the appropriate treatment for worsening signs and symptoms of COPD. The following are some rules of thumb for when to get help:

- Call immediately if disorientation, confusion, slurring of speech, or sleepiness occurs during an acute respiratory infection.

> **Action plan**
> a written document that gives specific instructions on what to do if you feel you need to see a doctor in an emergency.
>
> *All patients with COPD should have an action plan to deal with worsening symptoms.*

Living with COPD

- Call within 6–8 hours if shortness of breath or wheezing does not stop.
- Call within 6–8 hours if shortness of breath does not decrease with inhaled bronchodilator treatments 1 hour apart.

Do not wait longer than 24 hours to call your physician if you notice any of these severe symptoms:

- A persistent change in color, thickness, odor, or amount of sputum
- Ankle swelling lasting after a night of sleeping with your feet up
- Awakening short of breath more than once a night
- Fatigue lasting more than 1 day

34. If I'm having trouble breathing, do I need to wait for my doctor to return my call, or can I start treatment myself?

Severe respiratory symptoms are a life-threatening emergency. Early and aggressive treatment is recommended by experts. You are the one who can first tell if you are starting to get short of breath. Therefore, you are the one who can react the quickest to this warning sign.

You should discuss with your doctor what medications you should take when you first start to get short of breath.

You should discuss with your doctor what medications you should take when you first start to get short of breath. A written list of medications and dosages should be approved by your doctor and stored with your medications. This should be part of every COPD patient's "action plan" for treatment of exacerbations. You should always have a supply of all necessary medications handy so you do not have to wait to get them from a pharmacy in an emergency. Your medications may include bronchodilators, like **Alupent** or ipratropium; corticosteroids, like prednisone; oxygen; or even antibiotics. Some doctors recommend that people with frequent COPD exacerbations keep a supply of antibiotic medications at home to take right away if they develop early signs of an exacerbation, such as increased cough and discolored sputum.

Cecil's comment:

Another tip that might be worth remembering: caffeine can be used in extreme emergencies to assist in relieving extreme shortness of breath while you are waiting to see the doctor.

34. What is a "COPD action plan"?

Every patient with COPD should have an action plan for getting emergency care quickly in the event of severe symptoms. The action plan should consist of the following:

Things you will need at home:

- Contact information for doctor, hospital, therapists, pharmacists, ambulance, friends, or family that can help in an emergency.
- Written directions to the doctor's office, clinic, or hospital. You may not be able to talk easily, so giving directions will be difficult.
- Information on when to call the doctor, under what circumstances, and how frequently.
- A schedule of medications and what dosages to take under specific circumstances.
- Some method on how to assess whether you are improving.

Alupent

a brand name for the medication metaproterenol sulfate, an inhaled bronchodilator of the beta agonist group.

Living with COPD

- List of signs or symptoms that should prompt an immediate visit to the doctor's office.
- List of signs or symptoms that should prompt an immediate call for an ambulance and visit to the emergency department.

Things you will need if you go to the doctor's office or hospital:

- Complete list of your medications and dosages (prescription and over-the-counter), vitamins, and inoculations, as well as the name of the prescribing doctor.
- List of any alternative medicine treatments, such as herbal cures, homeopathic treatments, teas, or culturally based treatments (e.g., acupuncture, cupping, or coin rolling).
- List of all medications or other known substances to which you have allergic reactions.
- Copies of your most recent electrocardiogram, PFT, spirometric results, or similar tests/reports.
- Some cash to spend.
- Updated copy of your advanced directive, medical proxy, or medical power of attorney form and organ donation card, if applicable.
- Description of your medical history, in chronological sequence (including your use of tobacco, alcohol, or drugs).
- Insurance company cards or at least their names and policy numbers.
- Names, addresses, and phone numbers of your next of kin.

This action plan should be developed with the help of your physician, after a full assessment of the following:

- Availability and response times of ambulances
- Availability of friends and family who can drive in an emergency
- Nearness to an emergency room or doctor's office
- Availability of relatives or friends who can stay with you until you improve or a visit to the doctor is decided on

After this assessment, you can develop an action plan with your doctor and determine the appropriate treatment steps for signs and symptoms of respiratory difficulty. Family members and those who are close to you should be informed and participate in this emergency action plan.

Cecil's comment:

I developed a system that I have used with great success. I have a standard student notebook with a red cross stenciled on the front of it. Inside, I have the following information organized into different sections of the book:

- *TAB A = All personal information, such as address, telephone number, and emergency contact information.*
- *TAB B = Copy of my durable power of attorney and pertinent insurance documents and phone number of preferred hospital, as well as telephone numbers and names of all medical providers and pharmacy that I use.*
- *Tab C = List of all medications, including time of dosage, prescription numbers, prescribing doctor's name and telephone number; a list of all illnesses that have been diagnosed and the dates of diagnosis; and a list of allergies and drug interactions.*
- *Tab D = Family medical history and dates and reasons for family deaths. Siblings' names, telephone numbers,*

and medical history, as well as their current ongoing medical problems.

- *Tab E = Copies of results of all tests or procedures performed within the past year and name and telephone number of the attending physician.*
- *Tab F = Miscellaneous notes that pertain to anything that can't be placed in a particular area of interest, for example, number of years I smoked and my quitting date, how much I smoked, and the last date I was admitted to the hospital and for what reason.*
- *Tab G = Blank notebook paper on which to write the doctor's advice to me from the last visit or questions I want to ask him on my next visit.*

I notified my local ambulance company of this notebook and its location to ensure that it is always with me if I am incapacitated. This notebook is never far from me; I take it with me any time I leave the house for any reason. When I am at home, I have it by my bedside.

35. What are advance directives and why do I need them?

Advanced directive

your oral and written instructions about your future medical care, in the event that you become unable to speak for yourself.

Advance directive is a general term that refers to your oral (spoken) and written instructions about your future medical care, in the event that you become unable to speak for yourself. Each state regulates the use of advance directives differently. There are two types of advance directives: a living will and a medical power of attorney.

Advance directives give you a voice in decisions about your medical care when you are unconscious or too ill to communicate. As long as you are able to express your own decisions, your advance directives are not used, and you can accept or refuse any medical treatment. However, if you become seriously ill, you may lose the ability to participate in decisions about your own treatment.

36. What is a living will?

A **living will** is a type of advance directive in which you put in writing your wishes about medical treatment should you be unable to communicate at the end of life. Your state law may define when the living will goes into effect and may limit the treatments to which the living will applies. Your right to accept or refuse treatment is protected by constitutional and common law.

37. What is a medical power of attorney?

A **medical power of attorney** (also known as a durable power of attorney for health care, an appointment of a health care agent, or a health care proxy) is a document that enables you to appoint someone you trust to make decisions about your medical care if you cannot make those decisions yourself. The person you appoint may be called your health care agent, surrogate, attorney-in-fact, or proxy. In many states, the person you appoint through a medical power of attorney is authorized to speak for you any time that you are unable to make your own medical decisions, not only at the end of life.

Cecil's comment:

I have a medical power of attorney. But, before taking this action, I discussed my decision with my family and assured them that I had complete trust in the individual I appointed.

Living will

a type of advance directive in which you put in writing your wishes about medical treatment should you be unable to communicate at the end of life.

Your right to accept or refuse treatment is protected by constitutional and common law.

Medical power of attorney

a document that enables you to appoint someone you trust to make decisions about your medical care if you cannot make those decisions yourself.

39. Are there things I <u>shouldn't do</u> when my breathing gets worse?

Although there are many effective measures you can take at home to treat increased signs and symptoms, there are also actions that should be avoided. If you do any of the following, it can make your condition worse:

- Do not take any extra doses of any medication that you have not discussed first with your doctor in your emergency action plan. This is especially true of theophylline—overdoses of theophylline can lead to seizures.
- Do not take alcohol or any medication that may suppress your breathing. Medications that can suppress your breathing include codeine or any other cough suppressant, prescription pain killers, sedatives, and sleep aids.
- Do not increase the liter flow of prescribed oxygen unless you discuss this first with your physician.
- Do not smoke or inhale secondary smoke. Avoid dusting, wearing perfumes, and being near fumes from fresh paint or cleaning solutions.
- Do not wait any longer than 24 hours to contact your doctor if symptoms continue.

40. What is an "exacerbation" of COPD?

Exacerbation

an increase in the severity of the signs or symptoms of a disease.

An **exacerbation** of COPD is a rapid, sometimes sudden, and prolonged worsening of a patient's cough, an increased amount of mucus, and a worsening of the shortness of breath. Wheezing is often increased or noted for the first time. Exacerbations are often caused by bronchial infections; however, fever is uncommon. These exacerbations often are life threatening and can lead to hospitalization. Often, the patient needs the mechanical support of a ventilator until the acute symptoms have resolved. Unfortunately, some patients do not recover sufficiently from the acute episode to enable them to breathe on their own. There is no way of knowing who will improve and who will not after such an episode. A person with COPD may initially have one or two acute exacerbations per year, which resolve readily with treatment, and many people recover and return to the same level of functioning they had before the exacerbation. The number of exacerbations per year and the severity of exacerbations can increase as the diseases progresses.

A COPD exacerbation is a medical emergency that requires the immediate attention of a doctor.

41. What are the causes of a COPD exacerbation?

There are two very common causes of COPD exacerbations:

- Lung infections, such as bronchitis and pneumonia. Infections are the most common cause of COPD exacerbations and are usually caused by a virus, but they can also be caused by bacteria.
- Lung irritation from dust, fumes, and other sources of air pollution.

When you experience a COPD exacerbation, there is a dramatic increase in mucus production in your lungs as well as a narrowing of the airways of the lungs (bronchial tubes). The increased mucus production and airway narrowing decrease the air flow in the lungs, worsening the symptoms of cough and shortness of breath.

Other causes of COPD exacerbations include heart failure, allergic reactions, accidental inhalation of food or stomach contents into the lungs, and exposure to temperature changes or chemicals. In about one third of COPD exacerbations, doctors cannot find a cause.

The symptoms of a COPD exacerbation are a sudden worsening of your usual symptoms, including

- Increased shortness of breath and wheezing
- Increased cough with or without sputum (mucus), and a change in the color or amount of the sputum

Fever, insomnia, fatigue, depression, and confusion may also be present.

42. How is a COPD exacerbation treated?

How the doctor treats your COPD exacerbation depends on how severe it is. You may have to visit your doctor's office or go to an outpatient clinic, or you may even have to be admitted to the hospital for treatment.

Doctors usually use the following medications to treat COPD exacerbations:

Bronchodilator

a medication that increases the caliber of the airways of the lungs and makes it easier to breathe.

Ipratropium bromide

an inhaled, short-acting, anticholinergic bronchodilator.

Corticosteroids

hormones that are naturally produced by the adrenal glands of your body.

- *Bronchodilators:* these are medications that relax the bronchial tubes and make it easier to breathe. These medications may include inhaled anticholinergics (e.g., **ipratropium bromide**) and beta–2 agonists (e.g., albuterol).
- *Oral corticosteroids:* these reduce inflammation in the bronchial tubes and may make breathing easier. They are typically given for 5–14 days in those who

are not already receiving long-term therapy with oral corticosteroids.

- *Ventilators/respirators:* A ventilator is a machine that can help you to breathe if you are unable to get enough oxygen in your blood through your own breathing. This is used only if you are not responding to medication.
- *Supplemental oxygen:* oxygen is administered to increase the amount of oxygen in your blood. This may help reduce shortness of breath.
- *Antibiotics:* often used when a bacterial infection is considered likely. People with COPD have an increased risk of pneumonia and frequent respiratory infections. Although most infections are caused by a virus, some are caused by bacteria. Some experts believe that because most exacerbations are caused by viruses, antibiotics should not be used unless there is a demonstrated bacterial infection.

Cecil's comment:

The extended use of antibiotics can kill the "good" bacteria in your digestive system; these are necessary for the body to function properly. Prolonged use of antibiotics can sometimes result in diarrhea. Notify your physician if this occurs.

43. What are the warning signs of infection?

Although most infections can be successfully treated, you must be able to recognize an infection's immediate symptoms for proper and effective care.

- Increased shortness of breath, difficulty breathing, or wheezing
- Coughing up of increased amounts of mucus

Ventilator/ Respirator

a mechanical device for forcing air into the lungs of patients with respiratory failure; the terms ventilator and respirator are used interchangeably.

A ventilator is a machine that can help you to breathe if you are unable to get enough oxygen in your blood through your own breathing.

Supplemental Oxygen

a treatment in which an increased concentration of oxygen is made available for breathing, through a nasal catheter, tent, chamber, or mask.

Antibiotics

a medication, usually derived from a mold or bacterium, that inhibits the growth of other microorganisms. Antibiotics are used to treat infections by bacteria, such as pneumonia.

Living with COPD

- Chest pain upon coughing
- Yellow or green mucus (may or may not be present)
- Fever (temperature over 101°F) or chills (may or may not be present)
- Increased fatigue or weakness
- Sore throat, scratchy throat, or pain when swallowing
- Unusual sinus drainage, nasal congestion, headaches, or tenderness along upper cheekbones
- Difficulty talking
- Difficulty walking
- Blue lips or fingernails

If you have any of these symptoms, contact your physician right away, even if you do not feel sick.

44. What can I do to prevent infections?

The lungs of people with COPD do not work well when it comes to clearing their lungs of bacteria, dusts, and other pollutants in the air. When these airborne pollutants deposit in the lungs, they can cause inflammation or infections that may further damage the lungs. Therefore, it is important to watch for signs of infection and seek treatment if you have them. You should follow these steps to decrease the amount of lung infections you get:

It is important to watch for signs of infection and seek treatment if you have them.

- Avoid contact with people who have colds, influenza, pneumonia, and other contagious diseases.
- If visitors have cold or flu symptoms, ask them not to visit until they are feeling well.
- Avoid crowds or situations where you must come in contact with many people, especially during the influenza season. Wash hands frequently with warm water and soap. Hand washing is especially important after you have been around someone with a

cold or the flu as well as after you have been at a social gathering. Hand washing is recommended before preparing food, eating, taking medications, using a **nebulizer**, and after coughing, sneezing, or using the bathroom.

Living with COPD

Cecil's comment:

I always carry a packet of moist wipes in my pocket or bag. I use these occasionally when shopping or just handling objects in a store. They eliminate the need for constant hand washing and are extremely effective in killing germs. When shopping with a basket or cart I always wipe the handle before using it. Other products are available at the local pharmacy that come in small, squeezable bottles and contain antibacterial lotion. These can be used to clean your hands after you have contact with anything that might have germs on it (especially other people with coughs or colds).

45. What is "environmental management"?

When a physician speaks with a COPD patient about environmental management, the physician is speaking about changing the areas where the patient lives and works to make them safer and healthier. This may include cleaning the home, conditioning the air, re-moving pets, changing hobbies or even jobs.

People with COPD need to manage the environments that they can change and should avoid environments that they cannot change but pose a danger to their health. For example, patients with COPD should keep their homes clean and free from excess dust, mold, or mildew. Air purifiers and filters should be used to

People with COPD need to manage the environments that they can change and should avoid environments that they can-not change but pose a danger to their health.

remove dust from the air, and dehumidifiers should be used if the environment is wet or prone to mildew growth. When someone is cooking in the home, cooking fumes should be vented out a window or through a stove hood. Pets and other animals around the house can increase the amount of lung irritants in the environment from their fur, dander, saliva, urine, and feces. Patients with COPD should not have pets in the house. Heavy drapes and carpets can hold dust, mold, and other pollutants and should be removed from the homes of people suffering from COPD.

If you use breathing equipment, such as a nebulizer or an oxygen mask, to treat your COPD, the equipment should be regularly washed with soap and water. No one else should be using your equipment because that could result in the transfer of infections.

You should avoid outside environments, such as dusty work sites, farm settings, and automotive repair shops, that have high amounts of air pollutants. If you must enter or go near these sites, spend as little time in that environment as possible and wear a mask that filters out air pollutants. Your doctor can help you find a mask that is appropriate for you.

When the outside air is hot or humid or has a high pollen count, you should stay indoors in an air-conditioned environment. If the weather is very cold, you should stay indoors also or travel outside with a scarf across your face.

If you work in an environment that is heavily polluted or in a job that requires more physical effort than you can safely afford, you may benefit from vocational counseling and retraining for a different job.

Cecil's comment:

I purchased an inexpensive gauge that measures the temperature and humidity in my home. I have a small dehumidifier and a humidifier in my room and office area. If the humidity goes to extremes, then I go to my room or office and turn on whichever device is appropriate until the atmosphere in my house gets back to normal. For people with central heating and central air conditioning, you might consider talking to a service provider about installing a system on your unit that would keep the atmosphere stable in your home with the use of filters and built-in humidifiers.

The nebulizer is probably the most beneficial device that we can use as patients with COPD. It creates a mist when the air passes through the medication in the cup. The nebulizer and the **metered-dose inhaler** *are equally effective in delivering medication. The metered dose inhaler (also called an inhaler or a puffer) is a device used to administer a defined dose of medication for inhalation. An added benefit to the nebulizer is that the medications, which are in liquid form, are paid for by Medicare and most insurance companies and are the same as the MDIs and the diskus medications. This form of treatment should not be used to replace your MDI as a "rescue" when you are in an emergency situation unless this is supervised by medical personnel.*

46. How do I avoid the common irritants that cause shortness of breath?

The lungs of people with COPD are sensitive to certain irritating substances in the air, such as cigarette smoke, exhaust fumes, strong perfumes, cleaning products, paint/varnish, dust, pollen, pet dander, and air pollution. Extreme cold or hot weather conditions can also irritate your lungs.

Metered-dose inhaler (MDI)

an aerosol container that dispenses a fixed amount of medication for inhalation ("puffer").

You can avoid some of these irritants by

- Asking those around you not to smoke.
- Sitting in nonsmoking sections of public places.
- Requesting smoke-free hotel rooms and rental cars.
- Avoiding underground parking garages.
- Avoiding high-traffic or industrialized areas.
- Not using perfumes, scented lotions, or other highly scented products that may irritate your lungs.
- Using nonaerosol cleaning or painting products in well-ventilated areas and wearing a mask or handkerchief over your mouth when cleaning (dusting, vacuuming, sweeping) or working in the yard.
- Reducing exposure to dust by regularly changing filters on heaters and air conditioners.
- Reducing mold and mildew by using a dehumidifier.
- Using a room humidifier if you live in a very dry environment.
- Keeping pets out of the house, especially if you **wheeze**.
- Using an exhaust fan when cooking to remove smoke and odors.
- Staying indoors when the outside air quality is poor and pollen counts are high.
- Following weather reports and avoiding extreme weather. During cold weather, cover your face when going outdoors.
- During extreme humidity, try to stay in air-conditioned areas.

Wheeze

an abnormal lung sound associated with lung congestion.

HEPA filters

HEPA stands for High Efficiency Particulate Air. It is a type of air filter that removes even very small particles from the air.

47. What is a HEPA filter?

HEPA is an acronym for the words high-efficiency particulate air. **HEPA filters** are a type of very fine air filter that traps very small particles in the air. They can be attached to air purifiers, vacuum cleaners, and air conditioning systems, and they also have many industrial uses. When attached to an air purifier, HEPA filters reduce the concentration of very small airborne particles, including many allergens, such as pollen, animal dander, and dust mites. Keep in mind that air purifiers are designed to filter a specific amount of confined space. Therefore, you must know the dimensions of the room you plan to place the air purifier in when you go to purchase one. Air purifiers can be expensive and require that the filter be changed every 3–6 months.

An air purifier should be placed in a room where you spend a lot of time, such as the bedroom or living room. They are designed to run 24 hours a day, and that is how they should be used. The room should have the doors and windows closed so that the air in that room can be "purified."

An air purifier should be placed in a room where you spend a lot of time, such as the bedroom or living room.

Cecil's comment:

The HEPA filter is the most accepted form of air filter. I have used the ionizer type of air filter and found that it worsened my breathing problems. I did some investigating and found that anything with an ion generator is dangerous to our lungs because it produces ozone, which can irritate the lung linings.

48. Will an air purifier with a HEPA filter help my COPD?

This is a question that you need to discuss with your **pulmonologist** before investing in a unit. For patients with COPD who have allergies or asthma that might contribute to their exacerbations, an air filter helps decrease the amount of allergens in the air that they

Pulmonologist

a medical specialist in lung diseases.

breathe. Whether this results in a decreased amount of COPD exacerbations is controversial. This issue has not be examined closely in the medical literature.

49. My doctor has recommended that I see a vocational counselor. Why would I need to have a vocational counselor for my COPD?

COPD is a serious, progressive, and sometimes debilitating disease. By the time most patients are diagnosed, they have lost more than half their lung function and have a corresponding decrease in physical ability. Their job may expose them to pulmonary irritants or they may be unable to perform their work any longer. With these issues in mind, your physician may recommend a vocational counselor. The vocational counselor's job is to make sure that there is an adequate fit between you and your work. Assistance provided by that counselor may include testing your interest and aptitude for various jobs, occupational exploration, setting new occupational goals, locating the right type of training program, and exploring educational or training facilities that you may use to achieve an occupational goal.

50. Is COPD associated with sleep apnea?

Sleep apnea is a condition in which a patient stops breathing for a few seconds during deep sleep. The patient often wakes up during this episode, then quickly falls back to sleep. This disease occurs mostly in obese individuals and is thought to be caused by blocking of the upper airway by the tongue and soft tissues

Sleep apnea

a condition where the patient has pauses in breathing during sleep. These episodes can last several seconds to half a minute.

of the throat. Prolonged sleep apnea can result in excessive sleepiness, headaches, and heart and lung disease.

Sleep has well-recognized effects on breathing, causing slower, deeper breathing and increased resistance to inhaling in the upper airways, especially during rapid eye movement (REM) sleep. This slower breathing and increased airway resistance does not have an adverse effect in healthy individuals but may cause problems in patients with COPD. In these patients, slower breathing and increased airway resistance can result in low levels of oxygen (hypoxemia) and higher levels of carbon dioxide (hypercapnia) in the blood. Night time oxygen **desaturation** in patients with COPD is fairly common and is often unrecognized. However, this nocturnal oxygen desaturation is not usually caused by obstructive sleep apnea. Instead, it can be attributed to lung damage caused by COPD in addition to the normal effects of sleep on breathing. Thin patients with COPD who have normal levels of oxygen during the day and short episodes of oxygen desaturation during sleep rarely develop coexisting upper airway obstruction or "obstructive sleep apnea." However, in some obese individuals with COPD, an "overlap syndrome" occurs, adding an obstructive sleep apnea component to the typical mechanisms of low oxygen saturation in patients with COPD.

During the evaluation of a patient for obstructive sleep apnea, a doctor may ask about morning headaches and daytime sleepiness to help make the diagnosis. He may ask the patient's spouse whether he or she is aware of the partner's intense snoring or notice pauses in breathing followed by loud bursts of snoring when

Desaturation

a decrease in the amount of oxygen in the blood.

breathing resumes. Spouses often choose to sleep in a separate room because of it. These reports strongly suggest the presence of obstructive sleep apnea. The diagnosis can be confirmed in a sleep laboratory using a test called the polysomnogram. If obstructive sleep apnea is diagnosed, it can be treated with either a breathing device called continuous positive airway pressure machine (CPAP) or surgery. If the assessment reveals low oxygen saturation but no obstruction, the treatment is much less clear. Oxygen therapy is recommended by some; other scientists believe that it does not improve the patient's health.

51. What is endotracheal intubation?

Endotracheal intubation is performed in patients with respiratory failure. It is a life-saving treatment for patients critically ill with COPD. The **endotracheal tube** allows the patient to have a machine take over the work of breathing when they can no longer do it themselves.

Endotracheal tube

a flexible tube that is inserted nasally or orally or into a tracheostomy to pump air into the lungs.

The procedure itself can be performed in an emergency room, an intensive care unit, or even out of the hospital in severe emergencies at the home or job site. The endotracheal tube is a soft, flexible, clear plastic tube that is place either through the nose or in the mouth and advanced through the throat, past the voice box (larynx), and into the main breathing tube of the lung, called the **trachea**. Because the tube is placed through the vocal cords, while the patient is intubated, he or she is unable to speak. The tube extends from the mouth 6 or 8 inches and ends deep in the chest, just above where the main breathing tube of the lungs (trachea) branches into the two smaller tubes called the **bronchi**. The endotracheal tube is then secured in the

Trachea

the wind pipe or main airway that goes from the throat to the center of the chest.

Bronchi

the main wind pipe divides into to these smaller airways in the middle of the chest.

mouth with tape and connected to a ventilator by a flexible plastic hose.

Sometimes, the upper airway is blocked, and a tube cannot be passed through the nose or mouth. Alternatively, the doctor determines that the tube will have to be placed for a longer time than expected. In these cases, a tube can be surgically inserted through the neck and into the trachea. Placement of this type of tube is called a **tracheostomy**. The endotracheal tube serves three major functions. It keeps the airway open and does not allow the tongue, soft tissues of the throat, or mucus to block the air from coming into the lungs. It also allows doctors and nurses to suction the lungs of excessive mucus. Finally, and most importantly, it allows the patient to be connected to a ventilator, a machine that forces oxygen into the lungs when the patient is unable to do the work of breathing on his or her own.

Tracheostomy

an operation to make an opening into the main wind pipe in your neck (the trachea).

52. What is a ventilator?

The ventilator is a machine that is designed to provide artificial respiration for a patient with respiratory failure of any cause. The ventilator pumps humidified air (with a measured amount of oxygen) into the lungs via the endotracheal tube or tracheostomy tube. The elasticity of the lungs allows the air to be expelled. Ventilators are used to help control the amount of oxygen and the volume of air flowing into the lungs. In the hospital, ventilators are carefully monitored and adjusted only by people who are qualified to do so; these include respiratory therapists, nurses, and doctors.

Ventilators are very effective at treating respiratory failure, but they are not without their problems. For example, ventilators may interfere with the patient's ability to communicate and swallow. Ventilators can increase the blood levels of oxygen and decrease carbon dioxide levels, but they do not reverse the underlying disease. Patients complain that it is very unnatural to have a machine breathe for them, and the endotracheal tubes can be uncomfortable. Therefore, many patients need to receive extra sedation while on the ventilator. In patients with very severe COPD, the patient may never recover enough lung function to get off the ventilator. Generally, those patients who have worse lung function and whose functional status is very poor are less likely to regain independent breathing. Finally, while the patient is using the ventilator, physicians need to take many blood tests and x-ray studies to monitor the disease progress and the efficiency of the ventilator.

Cecil's comment:

We are susceptible to having problems being removed from the ventilator/respirator in some cases. It is a good idea to talk to other people who have had experiences with the ventilator before your operation or procedure. The doctor can explain to you what will happen, but most of the time, they have not experienced it. A person with the actual experience can give you a much better idea of what to expect and could cut down on nervousness and anxiety.

53. How do I make the most of my visit with my doctor?

Studies have shown that patients who are involved in their own treatment plan are much more likely to comply with it. Further, when the patient collaborates with the doctor, he or she gains a sense of control over the illness, and that control increases the patient's sense of well being and quality of life. If each patient with COPD takes an active role in the management of his or her disease, he or she can expect to achieve optimal results from medications and therapies and avoid the complications of secondary infections or the debilitating results of sedentary living.

See the checklist below. When visiting your doctor, you should review the items on the checklist to see whether you are on schedule for the appropriate tests, procedures, or treatments.

Checklist of Medical Tests or Procedures

Consult with your doctors and therapists to decide which tests or procedures should be conducted periodically (as appropriate to your case) and the frequency:

1. Tests recommended every 3 months:
    1. Blood pressure, pulse, temperature, weight, oxygen saturation
    2. Spirometry
    3. Blood tests for glucose, theophylline, and digoxin levels, liver function, and so on
2. Test recommended every 6 months:
    1. Electrocardiogram
    2. Bone density test
3. Tests recommended every year
    1. Mammogram
    2. Blood tests and stool samples for cancer markers
    3. Digital rectal examination
    4. Prostate examination

4. Flu shot, annually
5. Full pulmonary function tests every 2–3 years
6. Pneumococcus vaccine every 5 years

Cecil's comment:

The checklist listed below is a good one to use at your first doctor visit when you are initially diagnosed. I also prepare a list of my current problems and questions that pertain to my current problems.

Questions To Ask Your Doctor during your regular visit:

(This is a suggested list of questions—add your own to the list if desired.)

1. *What is my diagnosis and how can I learn more about it?*
2. *What areas of my body can be affected by my condition? How?*
3. *What tests will you use to diagnose my problem? How safe are these tests?*
4. *What is the likely course of my problem? What is the long-term outlook?*
5. *What are my treatment options? Do I take treatments regularly or as needed?*
6. *What can I do on my own to improve my condition?*
7. *I have certain special concerns (e.g., exercise, travel, work environment, certain foods, pets, pregnancy, surgery, alternative medicines, relative with serious outcomes with similar disease or medications). How do these issues relate to my condition?*
8. *Regarding my medications, how much do I take and for how long? What does this medication do and when will I feel/know that they are working? What are the*

possible side effects of the medications and how should we monitor for them (e.g., laboratory testing, blood pressure reading)? Will these medications interact with the other medications that I am taking? What happens if I forget to take it?

9. *If my symptoms worsen, what should I do on my own? When should I call your office versus going to the emergency room? What should I do late at night?*

10. *Ask about developing a COPD action plan in writing.*

Remember: Prepare answers ahead of time for the "routine" questions that doctor will ask. Prepare your own list of questions for the doctor, in writing. Bring a copy of your medical records, if you have been seen by other specialists in the past. Bring a list of medications that you have tried in the past and those you are currently using. Establishing an accurate diagnosis is essential for proper treatment. You become the most important person in this process by accurately describing to your doctor the character, location, duration, and time of onset of your symptoms. You should also inform your doctor about vitamins, herbs, and medications you are taking. For example, long-term use of certain vitamins and nonprescription medications may cause abnormal liver test results; magnesium-containing antacids and supplements may be causing your diarrhea; and certain blood pressure pills can be the reason for constipation.

Request copies of the results of all tests that are performed. This allows quick access by emergency personnel if you are incapacitated or in a state of agitation or mental disorder. If you have a scheduled appointment for any of these tests, it is a good idea to not eat anything after midnight the day before. In some cases, the staff who schedule these appointments forget to tell you this information, and the test may be flawed or postponed.

PART FIVE

Smoking and COPD

I've been smoking for 30 years and have already been diagnosed with COPD. Isn't the damage already done? Do I have to quit smoking?

How do I stop smoking?

More ...

54. I've been smoking for 30 years and have already been diagnosed with COPD. Isn't the damage already done? Do I have to quit smoking?

Smokers with COPD experience a decrease in lung function that is much faster than the decrease in lung function that typically occurs with old age. When a smoker with COPD stops smoking, the rapid decrease in lung function tends to level off, so no matter how bad your lung function is now, when you continue to smoke, you make it worse. Small decreases in lung function may make a big difference in your ability to function. For example, it may mean the difference between dancing at your daughter's wedding and watching from the sidelines.

There are many reasons for you to stop smoking, even if it is difficult. Although COPD is not an inevitable complication of smoking, it is very common complication. If COPD is detected early, there are things you can do to slow its progression and preserve your health. Many patients who have COPD do not realize it. In fact, a study conducted by the **CDC** found that at least two thirds of patients with lung disease do not know they have it. Unfortunately, most people are diagnosed with COPD only after they come to the hospital with severe breathing problems for the first time. Of those who come to the hospital and require intensive care, 30% die in the first year.

CDC

Center for Disease Control. A division of the National Institute of Health.

The National Lung Health Education Program recommends spirometry (a quick painless test of lung function) for all smokers older than 45 years and for any smoker with respiratory symptoms, such as chronic cough, increased sputum production, or shortness of breath on mild exercise.

In December 2004, a study was published by the *Nicotine & Tobacco Research Journal* that alarmed physicians. This new US survey suggested that despite years of consumer education in print and television advertisements and in-office patient education, the great majority of smokers are misinformed about the health risks of their habit.

Researchers found that although 94% of the 1046 adult smokers they surveyed believed that they were adequately informed about the dangers of smoking, many either did not know the answer or answered incorrectly when asked specific questions about those health risks. Most importantly, they did not know that smoking increased their risk for developing heart disease, cancer, and COPD.

The survey also found a high degree of confusion when it came to "low-tar" and "light" cigarettes— products that have been heavily criticized because of the suggestion by their manufacturers that they are "safer," even though research has not shown them to lower smoking-related disease risk. About two thirds of the survey respondents indicated they thought these products were less harmful than regular cigarettes.

In light of this information, it seems appropriate to state the risks of smoking here, so that at least everyone reading this book is informed. Facts you should know include:

- Smoking cessation is essential in preventing and slowing the progression of COPD. In fact, the US

Surgeon General has stated, "Smoking cessation represents the single most important step that smokers can take to enhance the length and quality of their lives."

- Tobacco use is the leading cause of preventable deaths in the United States, claiming 430,000 lives annually. In fact, smoking causes more deaths each year than alcohol, auto accidents, homicide, suicide, and AIDS combined!

Smoking causes more deaths each year than alcohol, auto accidents, homicide, suicide, and AIDS combined!

- Based on data collected from 1995 to 1999, the CDC recently estimated that adult male smokers lost an average of 13.2 years of life and female smokers lost 14.5 years of life because of smoking.
- 85% of lung cancer is caused by smoking.
- 90% of COPD is caused by smoking.
- Using smokeless tobacco in any form (including chewing tobacco or snuff) is dangerous and can also lead to addiction and serious health conditions, like mouth, throat, and larynx cancer.
- Herbal cigarettes only switch one supply of tar and carbon monoxide for another. Herbal cigarettes are not a healthy substitute for cigarettes.
- Although nicotine can be dangerous to your health, the real danger in cigarettes is *not* nicotine, but the thousands of toxins present in tobacco and its combustion products, that are responsible for the vast majority of tobacco-caused disease.
- Cigarettes are *far more addictive* than nicotine gum or the patch, primarily because of the way in which they deliver nicotine. Therefore, these replacement therapies are helpful in conquering your addiction.
- Nicotine replacement therapy is safe for smokers, even if they continue to smoke. Replacing cigarettes with nicotine gum or patch is much safer than continuing to smoke.

- Switching to pipes or cigars does not decrease risks of smoking and in some cases may increase risks.
- Ex-smokers also enjoy a higher quality of life with fewer illnesses from cold and flu viruses, better self-reported health status, and reduced rates of bronchitis and pneumonia.

55. How do I stop smoking?

Physicians know that many smokers continue smoking, not through free choice but because they are addicted to the nicotine in cigarettes. A report by medical researchers in Britain found that nicotine complied with the established criteria for defining an addictive substance. Cigarette smoking, therefore, should be treated like an addiction. Like any addiction, stopping is difficult but not impossible. Successful smoking cessation is achieved through education, planning, and support from your physician, friends, and family. Quitting does not usually happen on the first try. Research scientists have found that most people try to quit seven times before they succeed, and unsuccessful quit attempts, although frustrating, are actually part of the process of quitting. For most people, the best way to quit is some combination of medicine, a method to change personal habits, and emotional support. The following sections describe these tools and how they may be helpful for you.

Quitting does not usually happen on the first try. Research scientists have found that most people try to quit seven times before they succeed

Get professional help. Your doctor has been trained to help you stop smoking. He or she can counsel you, help you chose from a number of quitting strategies, and even prescribe medication that can increase your chances of quitting for good. If have difficulty working with your physician, the American Lung Association,

Smoking and COPD

the American Cancer Society, the Will Rogers Foundation, and others offer courses in how to stop smoking.

Your doctor, dentist, or pharmacist can also direct you to places to find support. You may want to try a smoking cessation program or support group to help you quit—these programs can work great if you are willing to commit to them.

With the wide array of counseling services, self-help materials, and medicines available today, smokers have more tools than ever before to help them quit successfully.

Adding nicotine replacement to your smoking cessation plan doubles your success rate at quitting for good.

Quitting "cold turkey" is not your only option. Although some smokers are successful with this approach, medical studies reveal that adding nicotine replacement to your smoking cessation plan doubles your success rate at quitting for good. The most important element of the cessation process is the smoker's decision to quit—the aid or method of quitting is of secondary importance.

Talk to your doctor about other ways to quit. Most doctors can answer your questions and give advice, and they can suggest medicine to help reduce withdrawal symptoms. Some of these medications require a doctor's prescription; others can be purchased over the counter.

Join a Smoking Cessation Program

How do smoking cessation programs and support groups work? They help smokers spot and cope with problems they have when they are trying to quit. The programs teach problem solving and other coping skills. A smoking cessation program can help you quit permanently by:

- Helping you better understand why you smoke
- Teaching you how to handle withdrawal and stress
- Teaching you tips to help resist the urge to smoke

A review of smoking cessation products and services found that smokers are up to four times more likely to stop smoking by attending specialist smokers' clinics than by using willpower alone. If you cannot see your doctor, you can get some medicines without a prescription that can help you quit smoking. Go to your local pharmacy or grocery store for over-the-counter medicines like the nicotine patch, nicotine gum, or nicotine lozenge. Read the label to see whether the medicine is right for you.

Smokers are up to four times more likely to stop smoking by attending specialist smokers' clinics than by using willpower alone.

Prepare mentally for your quit date: you are not alone in your struggle against your smoking habit! Most smokers want to quit. However, it can be tough, and you will need lots of willpower to break the hold of nicotine—a powerful and addictive drug. Set a date to quit. Have other activities planned to help take your mind off smoking. Avoid people who smoke and places that are filled with smokers. In your mental preparation, it is helpful to make a list of all the reasons why you want to stop smoking. Place this list prominently in your home (e.g., your bathroom mirror or refrigerator door) to remind yourself why you are quitting. Here are some sample reasons to get you thinking:

- Better all-round health: stopping smoking reduces risk of 50 different illnesses and conditions.
- Heart attack risk drops to the same as that of a non-smoker 3 years after quitting.
- Cancer risk drops with every year of not smoking.
- Live longer and stay well: one in two long-term smokers die early and lose about 16 years of life.

- Set a good example to the kids (or other people's kids): you do not want to be a smoking role model.
- Have lots of money to spend on other things: smoking a pack a day can cost in excess of $1800 per year.
- You will experience improved fitness and easier breathing; you will be better at sports and climbing stairs will be easier.
- You have a better chance of having a healthy baby.
- Food and drink taste better.
- You will have better skin and complexion and no early wrinkles.
- You will have fresher-smelling breath, hair, and clothes and no more cigarette smells around the house.
- You will be back in full control and no longer craving or distracted when you are not smoking or unable to smoke.
- Travel on trains, airplanes, and buses will be easier.
- Work will be easier and you will not have to spend so much time outside or in the smoking room.
- You do not want to support tobacco companies.

Nicotine withdrawal may make you restless, irritable, frustrated, sleepless, or accident prone, but these things will pass and you will quickly start to feel the benefits.

Understand What to Expect When You Stop

Most people find the first few days difficult and, for some, it can be a long struggle, but things typically start to get better after the third or fourth day. Nicotine withdrawal may make you restless, irritable, frustrated, sleepless, or accident prone, but these things *will* pass and you will quickly start to feel the benefits.

Nicotine Withdrawal When smokers try to cut back or quit, the absence of nicotine leads to withdrawal symptoms. Withdrawal is both physical and psychological. Physically, the body is reacting to the absence of nicotine. Psychologically, the smoker is faced with giving up a habit, which is a major change in behavior. Both must be dealt with if quitting is to be successful.

Withdrawal symptoms can include any of the following:

- Depression
- Feelings of frustration and anger
- Irritability
- Trouble sleeping
- Trouble concentrating
- Restlessness
- Headache
- Tiredness
- Increased appetite

These uncomfortable symptoms can lead the smoker to again start smoking cigarettes to boost blood levels of nicotine back to a level where there are no symptoms.

If a person has smoked regularly for a few weeks or longer and abruptly stops using tobacco or greatly reduces the amount smoked, withdrawal symptoms will occur. Symptoms usually start within a few hours of the last cigarette and peak about 2–3 days later. Withdrawal symptoms can last for a few days to several weeks.

Deal with nicotine withdrawal. Nicotine is a drug found naturally in tobacco. It is highly addictive—as addictive as heroin and cocaine. Over time, the body becomes physically and psychologically dependent on nicotine. Studies have shown that smokers must overcome both of these dependencies to be successful at quitting permanently. You can roughly double the chances of successfully quitting smoking by using nicotine replacement therapies, such as patches or gum (Nicorette). The idea is to come off nicotine gradually by using a low nicotine dose to take the edge off the cravings and have a "soft landing." An alternative to nicotine products is the drug bupropion (Zyban), which is available only by prescription. Zyban is discussed in more detail in question 56.

Remove Cigarettes and Other Tobacco from Your Home, Car, and Work

Getting rid of things that remind you of smoking will also help you get ready to quit. Try these ideas:

Getting rid of things that remind you of smoking will also help you get ready to quit.

- Throw away all your cigarettes, matches, lighters, and ashtrays. Remember the ashtray and lighter in your car!
- Get rid of the smell of tobacco in your home and other places you smoke.
- Clean your drapes, carpets, clothes, and car.
- Have your dentist clean your teeth to get rid of smoking stains.

Do Not Use Herbal Cigarettes

Smokeless tobacco and herbal cigarettes also harm your health. These are not recommended as an aid to giving up smoking because they produce both tar and carbon monoxide. Some brands have a tar content that is higher than that in tobacco cigarettes. In addition, the use of herbal cigarettes reinforces the habit of smoking, which smokers need to overcome.

Do Not Use Other Forms of Tobacco Instead of Cigarettes

Light or low-tar cigarettes are just as harmful as regular cigarettes. All tobacco products have harmful chemicals and poisons. Some smokers switch to pipes or cigars in the belief that this is a less dangerous form of smoking. However, such smokers may incur the same risks and may even increase them, especially if they inhale the pipe or cigar smoke.

Consider the Money You Spend on Cigarettes

Smoking is expensive. It is not hard to figure out how much you spend on smoking: multiply how much money you spend on tobacco every day by 365 (days per year). The amount may surprise you. Now multiply that by the number of years you have been using tobacco and that amount will probably astound you.

Set a Date for Quitting

Set a date to stop smoking—any day will do—but choosing a date will help mentally prepare you for the task. Pick a date within the next 2 weeks to quit because that is not so far from now that you will lose your drive to quit. It also gives you enough time to get ready. Some people make a New Year's Day resolution, others pick their birthday, and you can join in with others on The Great American Smokeout (the third Thursday of each November). Think about choosing a special day:

- Your birthday or wedding anniversary
- New Year's Day
- Independence Day (July 4)
- World No Tobacco Day (May 31)

If you smoke at work, quit on the weekend or during a day off. That way you'll already be cigarette-free when you return.

Involve Friends or Family

If you live with someone else who smokes, it will be much easier to quit if you do it together. When expecting a baby, both parents should quit together. One common mistake is not to take the effort to quit smoking seriously enough. To quit successfully, you must make a sincere commitment to this challenge.

If Quitting Is a Struggle, Seek Out Other Treatments that May Help

Hypnosis, acupuncture, or other treatments may help some people, but there is not much evidence supporting their effectiveness. Use these treatments or services with caution; beware of requests for high fees or claims of "cures" or guarantees of smoking cessation. If you consider these to be aids in your struggle or a distraction from nicotine craving, then they have some value.

Find a (Temporary) Substitute Habit

Smoking also involves having something to do with the hands or mouth. Nonsmokers manage without this, so it is not necessary to have a long-term replacement for this element of the habit. However, if it is a large part of your smoking habit, you may need to deal with it. You may wish to chew gum; drink more water, fruit juice, or tea; or chew or eat something, in moderation.

Deal with any Weight-Gain Worries

Yes, it is true: many people (more than 80%) do gain weight when they quit smoking. The possibility of weight gain is often of particular concern to those who want to give up smoking. Nicotine changes the appetite and the body's energy use (metabolism). However, for a smoker who quits, the long-term weight gain is an average of only 6–8 lbs. Keep in mind that this weight gain occurs without the person trying to diet or add extra exercise to his or her daily regimen. Further, this weight gain presents a minor health risk when compared with the risk of continued smoking. In addition, improved lung function and some of the other health benefits of giving up smoking are likely to make exercise both easier and more beneficial.

Watch Out for Relapse

You will need to be on your guard against relapse, especially in the first few days and weeks after quitting smoking. "I'll have just one, it can't hurt" is the top of a long and slippery slope. If you are upset or under pressure, it is really important to fight off the temptation to smoke—do not let this be an excuse for slipping back. You could lose everything you have achieved just in a momentary lapse.

56. What are smoking cessation aids?

Unfortunately, smoking cessation medications are not commonly used by smokers. The vast majority of smokers attempt to quit smoking on their own, even though unaided quitting has a very high failure rate when compared with other strategies. It is hoped that with the help of their physicians, patients can use the effective medications that are available and quit smoking for good.

Medication

Bupropion hydrochloride (Zyban) is an effective smoking cessation medication. Although Zyban is proven to be effective, as with all drugs, there is a risk of side effects, and you will need to discuss with your doctor whether this form of therapy is suitable for you. Ideally, the use of such a medication should be accompanied by counseling, which some drug manufacturers provide by means of a toll-free line.

Zyban, which is also marketed as an antidepressant, was approved for use as a stop-smoking medication in the form of a sustained-release tablet. It works by desensitizing the brain's nicotine receptors and has shown promising results in clinical trials. The course of treatment lasts about 8 weeks. In one study, Zyban helped 49% of smokers quit for at least a month. In the same study, 36% of nicotine patch users were able to quit for a month. When both methods were used, 58% of smokers were able to remain smoke free for more than a month.

Zyban is available only by prescription under medical supervision. The drug is safe for most healthy adults, but there are side effects, the most serious of which is the risk of seizures (i.e., fits or convulsions). Therefore, Zyban should not be used by patients with seizure disorders, and it is not recommended for those with a current or prior diagnosis of bulimia or anorexia nervosa. This risk is estimated to be less than 1 in 1000, but other less serious side effects, such as insomnia, nightmares, dry mouth, and headaches, are more common. An independent review by the Consumers' Association concluded that "when used in a specialist setting and in conjunction with regular counseling, bupropion is at least twice as effective as placebo in helping patients to stop smoking."

Nicotine Replacement Therapy

Nicotine replacement therapies, such as chewing gum, skin patch, tablet, nasal spray, or inhaler, are designed to help the smoker break the habit while providing a reduced dose of nicotine to overcome withdrawal symptoms, such as craving and mood changes. Nicotine substitutes treat the very difficult withdrawal symptoms and cravings that 70%–90% of smokers say is their only reason for not giving up cigarettes. By using a nicotine substitute, a smoker's withdrawal symptoms are reduced. Now available by prescription, nicotine replacement therapy is clinically proven to be twice as effective as the cold turkey method. Nicotine replacement therapy eases withdrawal symptoms while the smoker gets used to not smoking, and the dose of nicotine is gradually reduced.

Nicotine replacement therapy deals only with the physical aspects of addiction. It is not intended to be the only method used to help you quit smoking. It should be combined with other smoking cessation methods that address the psychological component of smoking, such as is provided by a smoking cessation program. Studies have shown that an approach that pairs nicotine replacement with a program that helps change behavior can double your chances of successfully quitting.

Nicotine replacement therapy is available in many forms, allowing you to choose which would suit you best.

- *Patches:* Discreet and easy to use, patches work by releasing a steady dose of nicotine into the bloodstream, via the skin. Patches should be applied to a hairless part of your body, such as your upper arm, but they should not be applied to the same place 2 days in a row.
- The 16-hour patch works well for light-to-average tobacco users. It is less likely to cause side effects, like skin irritation, racing heartbeat, sleep problems,

Nicotine replacement therapies, such as chewing gum, skin patch, tablet, nasal spray, or inhaler, are designed to help the smoker break the habit while providing a reduced dose of nicotine to overcome withdrawal symptoms, such as craving and mood changes.

Smoking and COPD

and headache, but it does not deliver nicotine during the night, so it is not helpful for early morning withdrawal symptoms.

- The 24-hour patch provides a steady dose of nicotine, avoiding peaks and troughs. It helps with early morning withdrawal. However, there may be more side effects, such as disrupted sleep patterns and skin irritation.

- *Gum:* Nicotine gum is a fast-acting form of replacement that acts through the mucous membrane of the mouth. It can be bought over the counter without a prescription. It comes in 2- and 4-mg strengths. Nicotine gum allows you to control your nicotine dose. Learning to chew the gum properly is important—the idea is to chew gently until you get the flavor, and then "park" the gum in your cheek so that nicotine is absorbed through the lining of the mouth. Long-term dependence is one possible disadvantage of nicotine gum. In fact, research has shown that 15%–20% of gum users who successfully quit smoking continue using the gum for a year or longer.

The use of nicotine gum and nicotine patches together has not been widely researched nor has it been approved by the US Food and Drug Administration (FDA). However, existing studies appear promising. Smokers in most of these studies use the nicotine patches routinely (over 24 hours) and the nicotine gum as a "rescue," up to four pieces a day, without significant side effects.

- *Nasal spray:* This is the strongest form of nicotine replacement therapy and is a small bottle of nicotine solution that is sprayed directly into the nose. Absorbed faster than any other kind of nicotine replacement therapy, this can help heavier smokers, especially if other forms of nicotine replacement therapy have failed. The nasal spray delivers nicotine quickly to the bloodstream as it is absorbed through the nose. It is available only by prescription. However, the FDA cautions that because this product contains nicotine, it can be addictive. It recommends that the spray be prescribed for 3-month periods and not be used for longer than 6 months.

- *Microtab:* The microtab is a small white tablet that you put underneath your tongue and leave. It works by being absorbed into the lining of the mouth.
- *Lozenge:* The lozenge is like a hard candy or mint that you suck slowly. It gives you nicotine in a similar way to the microtab. This is the newest form of nicotine replacement therapy on the market. After undergoing the appropriate testing, the FDA recently approved the first nicotine-containing lozenge as an over-the-counter aid in smoking cessation. As with nicotine gum, the Commit™ lozenge is available in two strengths: 2 and 4 mg. Smokers determine which dose is appropriate based on how long after waking up they normally have their first cigarette.
- *Inhalator:* The inhalator is a plastic device shaped like a cigarette with a nicotine cartridge fitted into it. Sucking on the mouthpiece releases nicotine vapor, which is absorbed through the mouth and throat. Inhalators are useful for people who miss the hand-to-mouth action of smoking.

Nicotine replacement therapy is generally safe for everyone to use and certainly much safer than smoking. The US Agency for Healthcare Research and Quality Clinical Practice Guideline on Smoking Cessation recommends nicotine replacement therapy for

Nicotine replacement therapy is generally safe for everyone to use and certainly much safer than smoking.

all smokers except pregnant women and people with heart or circulatory diseases. If a health care provider suggests nicotine replacement for people in these groups, the benefits of smoking cessation must outweigh the potential health risk.

As you can see, there are many types of nicotine replacement. When choosing which type of nicotine replacement you will use, think about which method will best fit your lifestyle and pattern of smoking. Issues you may want to consider when choosing a type of nicotine replacement include the following:

- How much are you smoking now? Do you need a high dose of nicotine?
- Are your cravings worse in the morning when you first get up?
- Do you need quick relief from craving?
- Do you want/need something to chew or occupy your hands?
- Are you looking for once-a-day convenience?
- Do you need a rescue medication for "breakthrough" urges?
- Is your skin sensitive, and have patches given you a rash in the past?

Some important points to consider:

- Nicotine gums, lozenges, and inhalers are oral substitutes that allow you to control your dosage to help keep cravings at bay.
- Nicotine nasal spray works very quickly when you need it.
- Nicotine inhalers allow you to mimic the use of cigarettes by puffing and holding the inhaler.

- Nicotine patches are convenient and have to be applied only once a day.
- Both inhalers and nasal sprays require a doctor's prescription.
- Some people may not be able to use patches, inhalers, or nasal sprays because of allergies or other conditions.

PART SIX

Medical Treatment of COPD

What are bronchodilators?

Why do I need a flu vaccine?

More ...

57. Are there different levels of severity in COPD?

Yes, doctors divide COPD patients into three main categories: mild, moderate, and severe. This helps them to choose the right medications to treat the patient with, to predict and prevent complications of the disease, and to communicate details of the patient's medical condition easily with other physicians. The following describes the symptoms associated with severity levels of COPD:

Mild COPD

- The patient may cough a lot.
- The cough sometimes produces some mucus.
- The patient may feel a little out of breath after doing work hard or walking rapidly.

Moderate COPD

- The patient coughs more frequently.
- The cough is productive of more mucus.
- The patient is frequently out of breath after hard work or walking rapidly.
- Completing hard work or chores is difficult.
- It may take several weeks for the patient to recover from a cold or upper respiratory or chest infection.

Severe COPD

- The patient coughs even more frequently.
- The cough is productive of a lot of mucus.
- The patient may have shortness of breath during the day and in the evening.

- The patient may have shortness of breath at rest.
- It may take several weeks to recover from a cold or upper respiratory or chest infection.
- The patient can no longer go to work or do chores around home.
- The patient cannot walk up stairs or across the room without being severely short of breath.
- The patient tires easily.

58. How are patients with COPD treated?

COPD is a progressive disease that has many different treatments. However, not every patient with COPD requires all therapies. Physicians tailor treatment according to the type and the severity of the patient's symptoms, that is, according to the level of their COPD (mild, moderate, or severe) (Table 1).

59. How are patients with mild COPD treated?

In COPD, there are two types of treatment, treatment of symptoms and prevention. With patients with COPD, quitting smoking is the first and most effective way to prevent the disease from getting worse. To prevent infections, it is important for patients with even mild COPD to get both an annual flu vaccine and a pneumococcus vaccine. For patients with wheezing and shortness of breath, a short-acting bronchodilator (e.g., **albuterol** [**AccuNeb**, **Ventolin**, and **Proventil**]) used four to six times per day is appropriate, or a long-acting bronchodilator (e.g., salmeterol) may be used twice a day.

Albuterol

a short-acting beta agonist bronchodilator.

AccuNeb

a bronchodilator.

Ventolin

brand name for albuterol sulfate, a short-acting inhaled bronchodilator.

Proventil

brand name for the medication albuterol sulfate, a short-acting inhaled bronchodilator.

Table 1

Severity of COPD	Recommended Treatment Strategies
Mild	• Smoking cessation • Influenza and pneumococcal vaccines • Short-acting bronchodilators as needed
Moderate	• Smoking cessation • Influenza and pneumococcal vaccines • Short-acting bronchodilators as needed • Long-acting bronchodilators • Theophylline • Inhaled steroids (controversial) • Pulmonary rehabilitation • Supplemental oxygen therapy (as needed) • Mucolytics • Expectorants
Severe	• Smoking cessation • Influenza and pneumococcal vaccines • Short-acting bronchodilators as needed • Long-acting bronchodilators • Theophylline • Inhaled steroids (controversial) • Pulmonary rehabilitation • Supplemental oxygen therapy (as needed) • Mucolytics • Expectorants • Lung-volume reduction surgery • Lung transplantation

60. How are patients with moderate COPD treated?

Like the patients with mild disease, patients with moderate COPD need to stop smoking, get their flu and pneumococcus vaccinations, and use a bronchodilator for wheezing or shortness of breath.

Patients with moderate COPD may also benefit from taking theophylline (e.g., **Theo-Dur**, **Uni-Dur**, **Theolair-24**). Mucolytic agents and expectorants can help to clear the airways of mucus or phlegm. If these patients find themselves with shortness of breath while sleeping or severe shortness of breath with minimal exercise, then supplemental oxygen may be indicated. Rehabilitation is indicated for those moderate sufferers who cannot exercise or who should not exercise without professional supervision.

61. How are patients with severe COPD treated?

Patients with severe COPD can use all the therapies used for mild and moderate disease, but they require supplemental oxygen and pulmonary rehabilitation. These patients may benefit for surgical intervention, such as bullectomy, lung-volume reduction surgery, or lung transplantation.

62. What are bronchodilators?

Bronchoconstriction (also known as closing of the airways) causes the symptoms of wheezing and shortness of breath in patients with COPD. Therefore, bronchodilation should be the first-line therapy for treatment of symptoms in patients with COPD. There are two different types of **bronchodilator**: beta agonists and anticholinergics. Although these are different chemicals and affect your lungs through different pathways, they both result in opening of your airways, or bronchodilation. Each of these two different medications comes in a short-acting variety and a long-acting variety. The short-acting bronchodilators relieve your symptoms quickly (usually within 5–15 minutes),

Medical Treatment of COPD

Theo-Dur
a brand of long-acting theophylline.

Uni-Dur
a brand of long-acting theophylline.

Theolair-24
a brand of long-acting theophylline.

Broncho-constriction
a contraction of the smooth muscle in the airways that results in narrower air passages and difficulty breathing. A common condition in people with asthma. It may also be present in lesser amounts in patients with COPD.

Bronchodilation should be the first-line therapy for treatment of symptoms in patients with COPD.

Bronchodilator
a medication that increases the caliber of the airways of the lungs and makes it easier to breathe.

but the effects last for only a few hours. The long-acting bronchodilators can take longer to relieve symptoms (15–30 minutes), but their effects last for a much longer time (12–24 hours).

For patients with stable disease, a long-acting bronchodilator should always be used first. Shorter-acting bronchodilators can be used when you have a breakthrough of shortness of breath or wheezing.

63. What are beta agonists?

Agonists are medicines that exert their effects by combining with places called "receptor sites" on surface of cells in body tissues. Albuterol, for example, attaches to the lungs' beta receptors. Albuterol then is called a "**beta agonist**." Beta agonists are medications that cause the airways in your lungs to expand. This makes it easier to breath. Beta agonists are widely used for treating COPD. Beta agonists are used for both short- and long-term relief of symptoms. Short-acting beta agonists work quickly (usually within 5 minutes) and provide short-term relief of symptoms of wheezing and shortness of breath. Short-acting beta agonists also may be used before exercise to reduce breathing difficulties. The long-acting beta agonist **salmeterol** does not work as quickly but provides up to 12 hours of relief. The long-acting beta agonist formoterol begins working quickly and provides up to 12 hours of relief. The side effects of beta agonists used at high doses are nervousness, irregular heart beats, and muscle tremors.

If palpitations and tremors are a problem for you, you may ask your doctor about a medication called **levalbuterol** (**Xopenex**), which is a type of inhaled beta

Agonist

medicines that exert their affects by combining with places called "receptor sites" on body tissues.

Beta agonist

a type of medication used as a bronchodilator in patients with COPD; not an anticholinergic agent.

Salmeterol

an inhaled, long-acting, beta agonist bronchodilator.

Levalbuterol

a type of albuterol sulfate that is formulated to have fewer side effects, such as tremors and rapid heart beats.

Xopenex

a brand name for the medication levalbuterol, a short-acting inhaled bronchodilator.

agonist that is formulated to increase the effectiveness of bronchodilation while decreasing the side effects of rapid or irregular heart beats.

Cecil's comment:

*Albuterol, the primary rescue inhaler, has side effects for some patients. It can accelerate the heart rate and can create anxiety attacks and cause severe "jitters." There is a substitute that can be used for this called Xopenex. It is reported to cause fewer palpitations and anxiety. It is currently available only in nebulizer form, but the FDA has approved an MDI to be released. The MDI **Combivent** is a combination of albuterol and ipratropium bromide. Some doctors prescribe this as a "rescue inhaler" for patients who cannot tolerate the beta-agonist inhalers.*

Combivent

a combination of two bronchodilators: albuterol sulfate and ipratropium bromide.

64. What are anticholinergics?

Anticholinergic drugs are an important part of COPD therapy and are considered by many physicians to be the first choice of drug treatment. Anticholinergics, such as ipratropium bromide (**Atrovent**), have been reported to produce greater bronchodilation than beta agonists at conventional dosages, although maximal doses of either agent may result in similar degrees of bronchodilation. Anticholinergics may produce bronchodilation in patients who have no response to beta agonists because they bronchodilate using a different mechanism than the beta agonists. The anticholinergics can also decrease phlegm production. In addition, they have minimal side effects, even in higher dosages. Ipratropium has a slower onset and a longer duration of action, making it more suitable for use on a regular basis; it has been shown to work as well as beta agonists in the treatment of acute COPD

Anticholinergic drug

a type of medication used as a bronchodilator in patients with COPD; not a beta agonist.

Atrovent

the brand name for ipratropium bromide, an anticholinergic type of bronchodilator.

exacerbations. Studies suggest that the newer anti-cholinergic drug **tiotropium** is also superior to ipratropium, as well as the long-acting beta agonist salmeterol, in terms of decreasing shortness of breath. Tiotropium demonstrated significant bronchodilation and improvements in lung function over Atrovent and requires only once per day dosing. Additionally, in a 1-year study, patients treated with tiotropium required fewer doses of rescue medications and required fewer visits to the hospital than patients who did not use an anticholinergic agent.

Tiotropium

a long-acting, inhaled, anticholinergic medication.

Cecil's comment:

It is our responsibility as patients to ensure that we inform our physicians of allergies and medicinal interactions. Atrovent is a prime example. If you are allergic to peanuts or soybean oil, then it is imperative that you notify your doctor to ensure that you are not prescribed Atrovent inhalers. Atrovent inhalers contain soya lecithin, which can cause allergic reactions in some people with peanut allergies. Complicating this problem, patients with peanut allergy can use Atrovent nasal spray or Atrovent inhalation solution because neither contains soya lecithin. If you are not sure, ask your doctor about a test to confirm that no allergy is present before you take the medication.

65. What type of long-acting bronchodilator is best, a beta agonist or an anticholinergic medication?

This is a controversial topic, and no single answer is right for everyone. Because the drugs work by different mechanisms, some people may have more relief from one agent than from another or may suffer more side effects from one agent than another. A volume of published evidence supports the role of long-acting beta agonists in the treatment of stable COPD. Long-acting beta agonists, such as salmeterol and **formoterol** given twice daily, can achieve enhanced air flow throughout the day and night. In cases when you need rapid relief of shortness of breath, a short-acting beta agonist, such as albuterol, with or without a short-acting anticholinergic (ipratropium), should be used for relief of episodic breathlessness.

The long-acting beta agonists (i.e., formoterol and salmeterol) are superior to the anticholinergic drug ipratropium

The anticholinergic bronchodilating drugs also have their advocates, and many physicians believe that every patient with COPD should be taking a long-acting anticholinergic drug like tiotropium. Early clinical experience suggests that inhaled tiotropium may be more effective than salmeterol in improving many characteristics of lung function. In a 6-month study that compared patients with COPD who took tiotropium with those who took salmeterol, the tiotropium group showed a better improvement in lung function, fewer episodes of shortness of breath, and better scores on the quality-of-life survey than the salmeterol group. Both inhaled medications reduced the need for rescue albuterol when compared with placebo.

If a single type of bronchodilator is not working, a combination of two medications can relieve symptoms, and this combination of drugs is frequently prescribed by lung specialists. Many studies show that combining the two drugs leads to greater bronchodilation than the bronchodilation observed with either agent alone.

Formoterol
a long-acting beta agonist that should not be used as a rescue medication.

Cecil's comment:

The MDIs do not have a counter on them for the number of doses used. The best way I have found to "keep track" of the usage is to estimate how much I use by employing a simple formula. I know that I use my Atrovent inhaler at a dose of three puffs four times daily. This means that I use 12 puffs per day. Because there is a total of 200 doses per canister, I can estimate when the canister will be empty by dividing 12 puffs per day into 200 puffs per canister and come up with 16 days. Now allowing for tests and clearing the canister when necessary, I drop the eight doses and change it twice monthly on a specified date. I take a piece of paper and write this date on it and tape it to the outside of the canister.

*Additionally, I use a **spacer device** when using my MDIs. The spacer connects to the front of the MDI, and it helps you use the MDI properly and ensures that the full dose of medication gets into your lungs. I start by exhaling all the air from my lungs. I then place the spacer in my mouth and make sure that I get a tight seal with my lips. I press the MDI and inhale slowly. If you hear a whistling sound, then you have inhaled too fast and may not have received the full dose of the medication.*

Spacer device

a mechanism to increase the efficiency of inhaled medications.

66. What are steroids?

Steroids (also known as **cortisol**, cortisone, corticosteroids, or glucocorticoids) are hormones that are produced in the adrenal glands of your body. The most common natural steroid, cortisol, is essential to your life and well being. When your body is under stress or has an illness, additional cortisol is released by the adrenal glands to combat that stress.

When made in a laboratory, steroids are a class of strong anti-inflammatory drugs that are used to treat a

Steroid

a general name for an anti-inflammatory hormone produced by the adrenal glands.

Cortisol

a steroid produced in the adrenal glands of the body that helps suppress immune function.

variety of severe inflammatory diseases, such as arthritis, asthma, and COPD. Steroids can be taken in the form of pills, as an injection, or, most commonly, as an inhaled medication.

Steroid medications are used to decrease inflammation and mucus production in the lungs and make them less sensitive to inflammation. Increased airway sensitivity and responsiveness are some of the main components of asthma.

Regular use of systemic steroids can result in substantial improvements in breathing for about one in five patients with COPD. Also, a modest additional number of patients with COPD report subjective improvement while receiving oral steroids despite not showing improvement on spirometry testing.

Some studies suggest that inhaled corticosteroids may both improve air flow and reduce the frequency and the severity of exacerbations for patients with moderate-to-severe COPD. Thus, it has become common practice to use inhaled agents in addition to beta agonists and anticholinergic drugs. The benefits of inhaled steroids in COPD are observed only when used in high doses.

An occasional patient has symptomatic and physiologic benefits from oral corticosteroids that does not occur with inhaled products. In these cases, it is important for the physician to use the lowest dosage possible. This dose is established by gradually reducing the dose of steroids over weeks to months until the patient again has symptoms; the dose is then raised a bit until the patient feels better. In some cases, benefits can be maintained even with alternate-day dosing.

Regular, long-term use of low-dose corticosteroids may slow the decline in breathing function in patients with COPD. More studies are ongoing to investigate this important topic. These studies are evaluating early, regular use of oral and inhaled corticosteroids to retard disease progression.

Corticosteroids should not be used in patients whose symptoms do not improve when they are used. The use of corticosteroids solely to slow the progression of COPD cannot be recommended until further data are available.

67. I've heard that steroids have a lot of bad side effects. Is that true?

Steroids can have side effects; however, the side effects usually occur with higher dosages or more potent formulations that are used over a long period of time (weeks to months). Most people who use steroids do not have side effects.

Thrush

thrush, a possible side effect of using inhaled steroids, is a yeast infection of the throat that causes white spots or a white layer on the tongue or throat.

Common problems related to inhaled steroids, especially the more potent varieties, are fungal infections in the throat called **thrush** and weakness of the muscles in the throat that can cause swallowing problems or a hoarseness of the voice. To decrease these complications, you should use a "spacer" with inhalation (or puffer) devices. After you use your inhalation device, you should rinse your mouth to wash out the medication that is left in your mouth and throat.

Long-term use of potent steroids, even inhaled, may pose risks for cataracts of the eyes, thinning of the bones (osteoporosis), and a decrease in your body's ability to make its own steroids (also called adrenal suppression). Indeed, if you take steroids for a long time, even inhaled steroids, your doctor may recommend that you take a larger dose of steroids before undergoing general anesthesia or surgery.

The body's adrenal system produces cortisol, and the brain monitors these levels in the bloodstream. The brain is unable to tell between the body's own cortisol and the cortisone from corticosteroid medications. Over time, a patient taking high doses of corticosteroids could develop adrenal suppression.

Adrenal suppression occurs in steroid users when the brain stops producing the body's own natural cortisol in response to increased levels of cortisone in the blood from steroidal medications. This becomes a problem if the patient suddenly stops taking his or her steroid medications because the body may not be producing its own cortisol, leaving the body much more susceptible to infections and illness. This is why it is so important to continue taking steroid medications of any type and not to stop abruptly. The dosage of steroids must be tapered off slowly under a doctor's supervision.

Adrenal suppression

a decrease in the body's production of adrenal steroids as a result of taking medications that contain these steroids, such as prednisone or hydrocortisone.

68. Are mucolytics helpful for patients with COPD?

A **mucolytic agent** is designed to liquefy the phlegm in the airways and make it easier to cough up. Mucolytics may be of modest benefit in patients with COPD. In a recent review of many studies on the use of mucolytics in COPD, researchers found that in subjects with chronic bronchitis or COPD, treatment with mucolytics helped reduce acute exacerbations a small amount and also helped reduce the total number of days of disability.

Mucolytic agent

mucolytic agents are designed to help loosen and clear the mucus from the airways by breaking it up.

N-Acetylcysteine

a type of medicine that may help move secretions out of the lungs and airways.

N-acetylcysteine (NAC) is the prototypic mucolytic agent, but because of its cost and limited utility, NAC use in its inhaled formulation is generally discouraged for COPD in the United States. By contrast, recombinant human DNAase (dornase), which has proven utility in patients with cystic fibrosis, has not appeared to help patients with bronchial disorders not related to cystic fibrosis.

Expectorant

a medication that helps one to cough up phlegm or mucus.

Expectorants are agents given to patients to loosen phlegm in their airways and help patients cough it up.

Guaifenesin

medication used to help clear mucus or phlegm from the chest.

69. What are expectorants?

Expectorants are agents given to patients to loosen phlegm in their airways and help patients cough it up. The most common expectorant is **guaifenesin**. Guaifenesin may lessen the stickiness of respiratory secretions, making it easier to expel them. Although unproven by medical studies, many patients report benefits from using over-the-counter expectorant drugs that thin mucus. For patients who continue to have difficulty due to chronic congestion despite optimal inhaled therapy, expectorants should be tried. Guaifenesin is available in a variety of compounds, and pseudoephedrine is commonly added. If you would like to lessen the side effects of pseudoephedrine, such as nervousness and tremors, you can ask for a formulation without it.

Theophylline

an alkaloid type of medication similar to caffeine that can cause bronchodilation as well as increased respiratory muscle contraction and endurance.

70. What is Theophylline?

Theophylline is a chemical agent similar to caffeine that is used as a bronchodilator. Theophylline is natural compound that can be found in tea leaves, although the theophylline used today is created synthetically in a laboratory. Before newer drugs, such as the beta agonists, were developed, theophylline was the mainstay of therapy for patients with asthma or COPD. Theophylline was found to act as a bronchodilator and cardiac stimulant. The role of theophylline in COPD management is somewhat controversial today. Although this drug does cause bronchodilation, it is less effective than the beta agonists and the anticholinergics. Additionally, there is a risk of serious side effects, such as irregular heart beats and seizures, if the patient takes too much of the drug. This has created further reluctance to use the drug among physicians and patients alike. However, for patients whose COPD symptoms are not well controlled on beta agonists, anticholinergics, and inhaled steroids, a trial of theophylline is justified. Introducing the drug slowly in escalating dosages may minimize some of the troublesome gastrointestinal or central nervous system side effects. In addition to bronchodilation, other potential benefits of theophylline include improved clearance of phlegm and increased force of contraction and endurance of the diaphragm. Because theophylline can be toxic at high levels, blood levels of the drug need to be frequently monitored by the use of blood tests.

71. What is the pneumococcus vaccine and why do I need it?

A **pneumococcus vaccine** is a preparation used to create antibodies to pneumococcal bacteria. When your body produces antibodies to a particular bacterium, it can prevent, or at least lessen, the effects of an infection with that bacterium. One study has found that the vaccine prevents pneumococcal infection in people with COPD, and many studies have demonstrated that the pneumococcus vaccine can lower the risk of complications that can result from pneumonia caused

Pneumococcus vaccination

used to prevent or decrease the effects of infections from pneumococcus bacteria.

by many types of pneumococcal bacteria. The pneumococcus vaccine is not effective at preventing complications of pneumonia caused by other forms of bacteria or by viruses.

According to the Advisory Committee on Immunization Practices, a pneumococcal vaccine is recommended for people who are older than 65 years of age or those aged 2 to 64 years who are at increased risk of getting pneumococcal pneumonia because of a long-term (chronic) illness, especially heart disease and lung disease. All patients with COPD should receive the pneumococcal vaccine and should be encouraged to be revaccinated every 5 to 6 years.

All patients with COPD should receive the pneumococcal vaccine and should be encouraged to be revaccinated every 5 to 6 years.

Influenza

an acute infectious respiratory disease caused by the influenza virus.

72. Why do I need a flu vaccine?

Influenza infections can cause an exacerbation of COPD, which may result in hospitalization. Many studies performed on patients with COPD have shown that the influenza (or flu) vaccine reduces exacerbations. In elderly, high-risk patients, there was an increase in adverse effects (mild fever and muscle aches) with vaccination, but these are seen early and are usually mild and not long lasting. Because the vaccine is made from only parts of the virus and no live viruses are used in the vaccine, **you cannot get influenza from getting the vaccine.**

73. I got a flu vaccine last year—why do I need another one?

Each year, a new influenza virus becomes dominant and causes infections. As a result, each year, the makers of influenza vaccines take the most common influenza viruses and make them into a vaccine. When you are inoculated with that vaccine, you are immunized against those viruses that the vaccine makers believe will cause the most problems. The next year brings a new dominant influenza virus, and you need to get immunized against it also. Influenza vaccines are recommended for patients with COPD every year.

Thoughts on COPD Treatment

As you can see, there are many types of medication to help people with COPD. Some can treat symptoms, others can prevent exacerbations. You should discuss your symptoms and your medical treatment with your physician. When your physician is provided with all the information about your symptoms, he or she can recommend adding medications or increasing doses to relieve your symptoms and make your breathing easier.

Medical Treatment of COPD

PART SEVEN

Oxygen Therapy for COPD

What is supplemental oxygen therapy?

When does a patient require oxygen therapy?

More . . .

74. What is supplemental oxygen therapy?

Oxygen therapy is a medical treatment for COPD and other diseases; with this treatment, an increased concentration of oxygen is made available for breathing. Oxygen is usually given through a nasal catheter, tent, chamber, or mask.

Oxygen therapy

a treatment in which an increased concentration of oxygen is made available for breathing, through a nasal catheter, tent, chamber, or mask.

When patients with COPD have severe disease, they cannot get enough oxygen to their body tissues (a condition that doctors call **hypoxemia**). Chronic hypoxemia results in severe shortness of breath, loss of energy, inability to exercise, difficulty concentrating, heart failure, and weight loss. Providing supplemental oxygen can increase the life expectancy of patients with COPD. When added to a pulmonary rehabilitation program, oxygen therapy can also improve quality of life. Some specific benefits associated with oxygen therapy include

Hypoxemia

a low oxygen content in the bloodstream.

- Improvement or complete reversal of cor pulmonale (the type of heart failure associated with COPD)
- Decrease in pulmonary hypertension, the high blood pressure in the lungs of patients with COPD
- Increase in body weight
- Reversal of polycythemia, the thickening of blood associated with COPD
- Improvement in intellectual function
- Improvement in muscle mass and exercise performance
- Possible reversal of sexual impotence
- Possible reduction in frequency of hospitalizations

Cecil's comment:

When your oxygen prescription is passed on to your oxygen supplier, the supplier assumes the responsibility to ful-

fill your oxygen needs as prescribed by your doctor. How-ever, some oxygen suppliers try to use the cheapest methods possible to meet the minimum requirements of the doctor's prescription. It is a good idea to discuss all your projected needs with your doctor when you are given a prescription. Then, have your doctor fill them out in detail. Remember, you do not want to sit at home all the time, so make sure that portable, lightweight units are included in the pre-scription.

75. When does a patient require oxygen therapy?

If your lungs are unable to provide your body with suf-ficient oxygen to work normally, you need supplemen-tal oxygen therapy. The criteria that doctors use when prescribing oxygen therapy is based on your history, physical examination, electrocardiogram, and **arterial blood gas** (ABG) results.

The ABG test requires the doctor to take a small sam-ple of blood from an artery in your body. The sample is usually taken with a needle and syringe from the wrist or elbow area. The blood sample is put on ice and sent to the laboratory for analysis. If your blood has a low level of oxygen (i.e., hypoxemia), then the doctor can order continuous oxygen therapy.

If you have other conditions, in addition to your COPD, such as pulmonary hypertension, right-sided heart fail-ure (cor pulmonale), or high red blood cell count (poly-cythemia or erythrocytosis), then oxygen therapy may be ordered, even if your blood oxygen level is not so low.

You need a prescription from a licensed physician before a supplier can deliver oxygen to your home.

If your lungs are unable to provide your body with suf-ficient oxygen to work nor-mally, you need supple-mental oxygen therapy.

Arterial blood gas (ABG)

a measure of the oxy-gen and carbon dioxide in the bloodstream.

Without a prescription, your insurance company is unlikely to pay for the oxygen therapy. The prescription specifies how much oxygen you need per minute and when to use the oxygen. Some people use oxygen therapy only while exercising, others only while sleeping, and still others need oxygen continuously. In the beginning, your physician will order several blood oxygen tests to determine what your oxygen level is and how much supplemental oxygen you need.

Cecil's comment:

*Some doctors test your need for oxygen initially with the use of **pulse oximetry**. If the result is above 90%, they would tell you that you do not need oxygen. Ensure that when this initial test is performed, it is with what is called a 6-minute walk test. This is accomplished by the doctor or nurse attaching an oximeter to your finger and actually walking until your oxygen saturation drops below 88% or you complete the 6 minutes without your saturation dropping below 90%. If you are already receiving oxygen, this same test can be used to determine the need to turn your oxygen levels up for exercise or exertion.*

When the doctor writes a prescription for oxygen, it is typically provided in one of three ways: oxygen can be delivered to your home in a cylinder of a gas, as a liquid, or through an oxygen concentrator.

Oxygen can be compressed into various-sized cylinders for ease of use. For example, oxygen can be provided in a small cylinder that can be carried with you or in large tanks. The large tanks are heavy and are suitable only for stationary use. The cylinders have a device attached to them called a regulator that controls the flow rate of oxygen. Because the flow of oxygen out of the cylinder is constant, an oxygen-conserving

Pulse oximetry

noninvasive measure of the amount of oxygen in the bloodstream.

device may be attached to the system to avoid waste. This device releases the gas only when you inhale and cuts it off when you exhale, enabling your cylinder to last much longer.

Oxygen can also be delivered as a liquid. Liquid oxygen is more expensive than the cylinders of compressed oxygen, but it takes up less space than the compressed gas cylinder, and you can transfer the liquid to a small, portable vessel to use when walking around. Liquid oxygen is very, very cold and must be stored in a container that is like a thermos. When oxygen is released from the container, the liquid oxygen converts to a gas and you breathe it in just like the compressed gas.

The final way oxygen can be delivered is through an oxygen concentrator. Concentrators are the most cost-effective type of oxygen delivery system. The oxygen concentrator is an electrically powered device that separates the oxygen out of the air, concentrates it, and stores it. Because you do not have to deal with deliveries, compressed gas is more convenient and it is a cheaper option than liquid oxygen. There are now compact oxygen concentrators that you can easily carry around with you so that you are not tied to your home like with the older units. The disadvantages are that you must have a cylinder of oxygen as a back-up in the event of a power failure. The electric company should be notified that you use the concentrator so that in the event of a power failure, they will work to get your service back as soon as possible.

Cecil's comment:

Some additional tips that are worth mentioning are the little "quirks" that go with an oxygen concentrator, the first being the humidifier bottle. When you clean it or refill it, ensure that the top is properly resealed. You can do this by taking the hose loose from the bottle and holding your finger over the outlet. The ball indicator should start to fall and the alarm should sound. This signifies that the bottle is properly sealed and that you are getting oxygen through the bottle. If you have a humidifier bottle, you should make sure that you have a water trap so that if the humidity between the concentrator and the interior of the house is different, the condensation turns to water and "floods" your nose. The water trap catches this moisture. Also, you should never use more than a 50-foot hose; the supplier should inform you that with anything over 50 feet, the output amount is unstable. It is also a good idea to ask your provider about a "liter meter"; this resembles a tire gauge and is used to check to ensure that the oxygen output is the same as the indicator on the concentrator.

There are several different kinds of concentrator units, and you should choose the model that fits your needs. For instance, the impulse type of unit requires no batteries and feeds oxygen only when you breath in through the nose. This is a problem with people who are "mouth breathers" or those with a deviated septum. The second kind of unit is the one that works on impulse when you breath but has batteries to assist in breathing if the breathing pattern is not consistent. The third kind has a constant feed from a liquid reservoir.

There are three typical ways of delivering oxygen. The first, and most common, is the nasal cannula. It is a two-pronged device, made of thin clear plastic tubing; it is inserted in the nostrils and is connected to tubing carrying the oxygen. The tubing can rest on the ears or be attached to the frame of eyeglasses. Although simple and inexpensive, the nasal cannula is an inefficient delivery method.

The second way to deliver oxygen is by mask. The mask is made of clear, flexible plastic that covers your nose and mouth. Masks work well for people who need a higher flow of oxygen and for those who want relief at night from the irritation of using the nasal cannula during the day. A demand-flow device can increase the efficiency of oxygen delivery. A demand-flow device senses the start of ventilation and delivers a pulse of oxygen during early **inspiration**, when it is more likely to be useful in gas exchange. Because patients with COPD inhale for approximately one part of the breathing cycle and expire for three to five parts, this method eliminates oxygen flow during expiration that would otherwise be wasted.

Inspiration
the act of taking in a breath, breathing in.

The third common way of using oxygen is via the transtracheal route. Transtracheal means that the oxygen tube goes directly into the windpipe in the neck (the trachea) and bypasses the mouth, nose, and throat. Placement of these devices requires an experienced physician, along with comprehensive support from a nurse or a respiratory care practitioner. The transtracheal catheter is held in place by a necklace. Because transtracheal oxygen bypasses the mouth, nose, and throat, a humidifier is absolutely required at high oxygen flow rates. Transtracheal oxygen delivery improves patients' adherence to therapy, and it enables the patient to receive oxygen continuously for 24 hours a day. Adherence is enhanced by the concealed oxygen delivery system. Exercise tolerance is increased, and studies have shown that the work of breathing is decreased. The transtracheal oxygen approach is often successful in patients who cannot increase their blood oxygen levels by using a nasal cannula. Reduced hospitalizations have been reported.

Cecil's comment?

I have found as a patient on oxygen 24/7 that the cannulas have some "quirks" that are worth noting. Be sure, as Dr. Quinn noted, to replace them very frequently. If they are used too long, they become hard and brittle, causing them to actually cut the skin and make sores in the nose. Also, they have a tendency to make sores over the ears when they are worn constantly. There are ways to prevent this. Ask your supplier about "ear wraps," small, round pieces of soft rubber that you slide over the cannula above the ears. I usually put a bit of glue on mine because there is no way to hold them stationary so that they do not move from over the ears. You can also obtain a cannula that has these made into the area above the ears. Also available is an extremely soft hose that is very pliable; unfortunately, it has a drawback in that if the slightest pressure is applied to the hose or cannula, the air supply is cut off. There are other things that are notable as well. When you are receiving oxygen, ensure that the nose stays moist inside. If not, drying will occur, which can create bleeding and sores. These can be prevented by using a non–petroleum based ointment and a saline solution, if necessary.

76. Is it dangerous to have oxygen in the house?

Oxygen is safe to use, and problems with its use are rare.

No, oxygen is safe to use, and problems with its use are rare. Although oxygen does not explode, it markedly enhances combustion. Therefore, you should never smoke while using oxygen and should warn visitors not to smoke near you. When using oxygen, you should stay at least 5 feet away from gas stoves, candles, lighted fireplaces, or other heat sources. Do not use any flammable products, like cleaning fluid, paint thinner, or aerosol sprays while using your oxygen. It is prudent to keep a fire extinguisher in your home and close to the place you usually use your oxygen. If you use an oxygen concentrator, notify your electric company so that you will be given priority if there is a power failure. Also, avoid using extension cords, if possible.

Maintaining and cleaning your equipment ensure good service and decrease your risk of infection. You should ask your medical equipment company that provides the oxygen therapy equipment to provide you with instructions on how to care and maintain your particular equipment.

Some general guidelines for your cleaning your equipment are as follows:

- You should wash your nasal prongs with a liquid soap and thoroughly rinse them once or twice a week.
- Replace nasal prongs every 2–4 weeks. If you have a cold, change them when your cold symptoms have passed.
- Your health care provider can teach you how to clean your transtracheal catheter and when to replace it.
- The humidifier bottle should be washed with soap and warm water and rinsed thoroughly between each refill. Air dry the bottle before filling with sterile or distilled water. The bottle and its top should be disinfected after they are cleaned.
- If you use an oxygen concentrator, unplug the unit, then wipe down the cabinet with a damp cloth and dry it daily. The air filter should be cleaned at least twice a week. Follow your home medical equipment

and services company's directions for cleaning the compressor filter.

Cecil's comment:

I have a sign on my front entry way saying "Oxygen in use CAUTION." In addition, I notify all my family and friends that the inside of my home is smoke free and also that they are not to use strong aftershave or perfumes when visiting me. If someone comes to my front door and I find that he or she has a strong odor or perfume, I politely ask the person to stay at the door because I am odor sensitive due to my compromised lungs. I have a patio table and chairs on my porch, and we converse there if necessary. I have a gas cook stove and was informed by my oxygen provider that it was relatively safe as long as certain precautions were taken. I reverse the cannula so that the hose goes down my back rather than over my chest. I do this by removing the cannula from underneath my chin and tightening it around the back of my head. I then clip the hose to my waist band or belt. This places me between the hose and the stove and gives me complete control. I also never lean over the stove. I always stand upright and arms length from the flame itself.

Oxygen therapy is not a prison sentence. With care and planning, you should be able to engage in many activities, including travel, without oxygen being an impediment to enjoying your life.

The easiest way to travel with oxygen is in your own car, van, or mobile home. However, you should still talk with your doctor, especially about the altitudes that you will be traveling to because your flow-rate prescription may need to be altered if you are going to a very different altitude. You will also need to arrange for oxygen refills in advance. When traveling by your own car or motor home, you have the freedom to carry your own portable oxygen equipment and to arrange for refills along the way. When transporting compressed or liquid oxygen, you must abide by some simple safety rules. The oxygen must be kept upright, away from heat and flame. No one should smoke around stored oxygen. Do not store oxygen in the trunk, where it can get very hot. Also, because oxygen containers release small amounts of gas periodically, keep a window partially open, regardless of the weather. When traveling on bus or rail lines, contact the operator beforehand and find out their policies on transporting oxygen. It is prudent to allow for 20% more oxygen than you need, in case of delays or emergencies.

When you travel by air, there are other things to consider. For example, even people with lung disease who do not necessarily use oxygen at home may require in-flight oxygen because the air pressure in an airplane cabin is lower during the flight than on the ground. You should discuss your travel plans with your physician, who can help you plan for your oxygen needs. It is also helpful to contact the airline's medical department and discuss your needs with them. If they can, the airline supplies the oxygen and other apparatus that your doctor deems necessary, but equipment may vary from airline to airline. Keep in mind that airlines have limited seats for passengers who need in-flight oxygen. Airlines may also refuse passengers who they consider to be unsafe to travel. Keep in mind that every flight includes lots of time on the ground, so you should allow for delays and layovers. Try to get a non-stop or direct flight to avoid extra fees and the hassle of arranging for oxygen on the ground if there are stopovers. Oxygen distributors should be able to provide this service.

You should discuss your travel plans with your physician, who can help you plan for your oxygen needs.

When traveling internationally, be sure to have the right electrical conversion adapters for your respiratory equipment. Liquid oxygen adapters with metric threads may also be needed. In many countries in Europe and Asia, oxygen suppliers are available to help you. Clearly, you should arrange for your oxygen needs in advance with a supplier who is experienced in handling international travelers.

Cecil's comment:

I have some additional "tips" from a patient's standpoint. I have been on oxygen 24/7 for approximately 9 years. When you are initially prescribed oxygen, the first thing you should consider discussing with your doctor is the supplier. In order to get the maximum flexibility for traveling and service, it is best to try and procure a nationwide provider service. If you do this, you do not have to have the problem of linking up to several providers and doing all the coordinating when you are traveling. You should also carry a prescription copy for oxygen with you at all times; this prevents problems if for some reason you need to get an emergency refill when you are away from home. You should also be familiar with safety procedures. When transporting oxygen, always transport it so that it is kept immobile. The danger is not an explosion but of knocking the head off the cylinder. I have personally seen a full oxygen cylinder go through a brick wall when the head was knocked off. I keep a spare underneath the driver's seat of my car. A small (B) cylinder is the perfect size to push underneath the seat with just a little pressure to prevent movement. As to flying, it is best to reserve a direct flight, even if you have to alter plans to some extent. For each "leg" of your flight, the airlines charge a fee. In addition, if you are on vacation and are traveling to higher altitudes than usual, it is a good idea to ask your doctor about a test that can be administered to determine the oxygen requirements at different altitudes.

It is also a good idea to notify your local fire department if you are on oxygen. This ensures that they keep enough emergency supply on hand in case of a prolonged power outage or storm damage.

A good way to store small cylinders is to get a soda case that is used for carrying 2-liter bottles of soda. This case can hold 6 (B) cylinders and keep them upright. You can usually get these cases at supermarkets, or some stores sell them as storage containers.

Oxygen Therapy for COPD

PART EIGHT

Rehabilitation for COPD

What is pulmonary rehabilitation?

Am I a candidate for pulmonary rehabilitation?

More ...

77. What is pulmonary rehabilitation?

Pulmonary rehabilitation is a program of patient education, as well as a carefully structured and closely monitored exercise classes. Pulmonary rehabilitation can improve a patient's exercise capacity, reduce shortness of breath, improve quality of life, and decrease the number and the duration of hospital visits for respiratory diseases.

Pulmonary rehabilitation can improve a patient's exercise capacity, reduce shortness of breath, improve quality of life, and decrease the number and the duration of hospital visits for respiratory diseases.

The classes in a rehabilitation program teach you about your disease, how to exercise, and how to accomplish more with less shortness of breath. The exercises increase your strength and endurance, allowing you to be more active and have less shortness of breath.

A pulmonary rehabilitation program is not a cure for your disease or a replacement for medication; however, it *is* an important addition to medical therapy.

The goals of COPD rehabilitation programs include helping you return to the highest level of function and independence possible, while improving your overall quality of life. Attaining these goals helps people with COPD live more comfortably by improving endurance, providing relief of symptoms, and preventing progression of the disease with minimal side effects.

Cecil's comment:

This is another area where exercise has to be re-emphasized. If the COPD diagnosis is made early, proper counseling should encourage the patient to become involved in an organized exercise program. This increases endurance and slows progression of symptoms.

78. *What are the components of a pulmonary rehabilitation program?*

When you begin a pulmonary rehabilitation program, you can expect the following types of therapies to be offered:

- Physical and functional assessment
- Exercise conditioning program
- Education program
- Occupational therapy
- Breathing training
- Psychosocial counseling
- Vocational counseling

All pulmonary rehabilitation programs begin with an assessment of your current disease state, your level of functioning, and your suitability for a rehabilitation program. The first part of this assessment is an interview. You will be asked about your symptoms, how well you are functioning, and what you hope to accomplish in the program. The interviewer will try to evaluate your knowledge about your disease and your medication. The interviewer will make a determination about your nutritional status as well as any anxiety or depression you may be feeling as a result of your disease. Finally, a physician will give you a thorough examination, administer lung function tests, and see how much you can exercise, either walking on a treadmill or riding a stationary exercise bicycle.

The rehabilitation physician will discuss the results of your assessment. Together with the physician, you can set the program goals both for increasing your knowledge base and for increasing your functional exercise capacity.

When you start the program, you will attend a series of classes and regular exercise programs, usually two or three times a week. The classes address the gaps in your knowledge about your disease and how to treat it. The exercise will begin slowly and will increase in duration and intensity, along with your increasing abilities. If you are using supplemental oxygen, your oxygen may also be adjusted to meet your needs at rest and especially when you are exercising.

In order to reach these goals, COPD rehabilitation programs may include the following:

- *Medication management:* A lung specialist (pulmonologist) will evaluate your current medications and adjust dosages or add new medications to achieve the maximum benefit. Oxygen therapy may be started to help you to exercise.
- *Patient education:* When you begin a rehabilitation program, you need to understand the program's purpose, the anticipated outcomes, and what is expected of you and your family members. The goal of education is to change your health beliefs and those of your family so that you can better accept the treatment plan and stick with it. Some examples of topics you will learn about during these educational classes include
  - What is COPD and how does it affect your lungs?
  - What do your medicines do?
  - How should you use your medicines?
  - When should you call your doctor?
  - How can you avoid infections and keep from being hospitalized?
  - How should you exercise and why is it important?

- How can you eat right and why does good nutrition keep you more active and out of the hospital?
- How can you conserve energy to accomplish what you want?
- What are the benefits of exercise?
- What is oxygen therapy and how does it improve your health?
- How can you cope with the limitations that COPD puts on you and your loved ones.

In the setting of group meetings, you will meet others with breathing problems and learn how they deal with their challenges. This gives you time to share your concerns and how you cope with living with breathing problems.

- *Exercise program:* Exercise training is the most effective method for improving your ability to perform activity. Exercises can decrease your respiratory symptoms and improve your muscle strength and endurance. Your rehabilitation specialist will design an exercise regimen that will accommodate your current functional status and accomplish your goals. An exercise regimen generally has four basic components: the mode, intensity, duration, and frequency of exercise. Some training programs involve up to twice-daily sessions. Lower-extremity aerobic training (i.e., training that causes you to breath hard for a long time) is the cornerstone of a reconditioning program, with an emphasis on building up your endurance and strength. You may also benefit from strengthening of your arms and shoulders. Other benefits of an exercise program may be an increase

Exercises can decrease your respiratory symptoms and improve your muscle strength and endurance.

in your endurance and an increased ability to perform daily activities. Because you will, ideally, continue this exercise program for the rest of your life, it is critical that you choose a mode of exercise that is enjoyable and convenient. In addition, you must have resources to continue this mode of exercise after you have left the program. Questions of what resources you need and how you can acquire them can be discussed with the program's case manager or social worker.

- *Breathing training:* Many patients benefit from breathing training, which decreases shortness of breath and increases the efficiency of your breathing. In some cases, it allows patients to regain control of their breathing, particularly in stressful situations. The two types of breathing techniques that are commonly taught are diaphragmatic and pursed-lip breathing.

  - **Diaphragmatic breathing** is taught when you are in a comfortable position, preferably reclining on a bed or chair. You will be instructed to place one hand on your upper abdomen and the other on your chest. You will be instructed to in breathe in deeply with a maximal outward movement of the abdomen. Once you becomes familiar with the method of diaphragmatic breathing, you can practice it while sitting or standing, or even while your at work. This method helps to reduce shortness of breath.

  - **Pursed-lip breathing** is a modification of the diaphragmatic method that can improve your oxygenation and reduce shortness of breath (called dyspnea by doctors). You will be taught to exhale slowly for 10 seconds against the slight resistance created by lightly pursing the lips. This

Diaphragmatic breathing

a type of breathing where the patient uses the diaphragm muscle rather than the chest muscles to breath in an out.

Pursed-lip breathing

a breathing technique used to decrease shortness of breath. Patients with COPD are taught to breathe in through their nose, and then on expiration pucker their lips together as though whistling (this provides back pressure and breathe out slowly through their pursed lips) which keeps the alveoli from collapsing before the end of the breath.

method slows your breathing rate and makes the oxygen exchange in your lungs more efficient. Pursed-lip breathing also creates a back pressure in your airways that helps to prevent airway closure and the trapping of air in the air sacks. About half of COPD patients can reduce their dyspnea using pursed-lip breathing.

- Case managers can offer you assistance with obtaining respiratory equipment, portable oxygen, and when needed, exercise equipment.

- Psychologists can help you develop techniques in stress management, relaxation exercises, and dealing with depression and anxiety, as well as offer emotional support. About 40%–75% of patients with COPD develop a reactive depression because their disease limits their employment, physical independence, sexual potency, social interactions, and self-esteem. Psychosocial counseling can increase a patient's self-esteem and also help family members cope with the patient's chronic illness. During your initial assessment, you should also undergo screening for major depressive illnesses that may respond to treatment with antidepressant medications and psychiatric therapy. Some patients have difficulty learning because of their educational or intellectual deficiencies (e.g., Alzheimer's dementia). Psychologists can test for this and determine the best way to teach the patient.

- Smoking cessation is an important part of any rehabilitation program. The physicians and counselors can help you quit smoking.

- Improving your nutritional status helps you increase your exercise capacity and helps you fight off infections. Dietitians can offer nutritional counseling in the program.

- Your COPD does not just affect you, nor are you expected to fight this disease alone. Patient and family education and counseling will help you and your family deal with the changes that COPD makes in your life.
- COPD can decrease your energy level and your ability to accomplish physical tasks. Vocational counseling can identify your work skills and assess your abilities. They can suggest energy-conserving techniques, such as modification of your work area, and can introduce you to devices such as electrical appliances and movable carts that you can employ to decrease the amount of energy you spend on physical labor. With this information, adapting to your work environment, retraining, or investigating new careers is possible.

To enroll in a rehabilitation program, begin by talking to your doctor about your interest in pulmonary rehabilitation. He or she can refer you to a program. If your doctor is unable to provide a referral, you can contact the American Lung Association for a referral to a program in your area.

COPD rehabilitation programs can be conducted on an inpatient or outpatient basis. Many skilled professionals are part of the pulmonary rehabilitation team, including any or all of the following:

Respiratory therapist

a professional charged with administering any of the therapies related to the respiratory system or breathing.

- Pulmonologist
- **Respiratory therapist**
- Physiatrist (an expert in rehabilitation and therapy)
- Internist (often the team leader and person with whom you continue treatment after the program is completed)

- Rehabilitation nurse
- Dietitian
- Physical therapist
- Occupational therapist
- Social worker
- Psychologist/psychiatrist
- Recreational therapist
- Case manager
- Chaplain
- Vocational therapist

Cecil's comment:

I have found that even patients with severe COPD can find ways to exercise, and it is a must in maintaining any quality of life. Regardless of your physical condition, every conceivable effort must be made to improve it. Pulmonary rehabilitation should be available to every patient with COPD. The muscles use oxygen when they work. If the muscles are deteriorated, then more oxygen is required for the muscles to be used. This in turn decreases the amount of oxygen that is available for the internal organs. It is also important to consult your doctor about referrals to a nutritionist for consultation on proper diet and vitamins.

Regardless of your physical condition, every conceivable effort must be made to improve it.

79. What happens after I finish the program?

It is expected that what you learn and practice during the program will continue in your daily life after the program ends. If you stop exercising after the program, the improvements you have made will soon be lost. The rehabilitation staff will work with you to design a long-term plan of exercise. The staff will guide you on how and when to exercise at home. Many programs offer a "maintenance" plan so that you can continue to exercise with others with breathing problems and be supervised by professionals.

80. Am I a candidate for pulmonary rehabilitation?

You should be considered for pulmonary rehabilitation when your lung disease begins to have a significant impact on your daily activities. To begin a pulmonary rehabilitation program, you must meet certain criteria. In most programs, you must be a nonsmoker or be willing to enter a smoking cessation program. Abusing other substances, such as alcohol, cocaine, or narcotics, usually makes you ineligible for a program. If you cannot exercise because of other diseases, you may not be able to participate in a program. Disease that might exclude you from a rehabilitation program may include heart disease, circulatory problems, terminal cancer, stroke, liver disease, or spinal cord injury, as well as advanced psychiatric disease or dementia. Pulmonary rehabilitation programs require a positive attitude and a willingness to work with the therapists. You also must be motivated to participate in both the educational and the exercise aspects of the program, and you must not have a mental illness that would interfere with your ability to participate in the activities.

Although lung function testing is part of the assessment of most programs, the results of theses tests are not used as entrance criteria for rehabilitation programs. If your lung function is reduced enough that you feel impaired in your normal physical activity and/or your job, you will probably benefit from a rehabilitation program.

Pulmonary rehabilitation programs have large treatment teams and use many resources. Therefore, these programs are expensive, although the costs can vary considerably between programs, depending on what the programs offer and where they are offered. If more than one program is available in your area, compare the costs and the services offered.

Even patients with severe disease and disability can participate in a rehabilitation program. Study results indicate that even patients with advanced disease can be successfully trained at maximal exercise levels. Even if as little as 10% of your lung function remains, you may benefit from an educational and exercise training program. By the end of a 3-week session, in some centers, a patient's ability to perform exercise may be doubled.

Even patients with severe disease and disability can participate in a rehabilitation program.

81. What if I'm still smoking? Will they let me into a rehabilitation program?

Current smokers may be eligible to enter a pulmonary rehabilitation program. Experts in lung diseases understand that smoking is a hard habit to quit. Rehabilitation programs include smoking cessation as one of their goals and offer programs in quitting as part of the rehabilitation. A minority of programs require that you stop smoking before beginning the program. Generally, if you are willing to try to quit, you will be able to find a program.

82. Will I be able to stop using supplemental oxygen after I complete my rehabilitation program?

Unfortunately, in most cases you will not, even after you achieve significant improvement in your exercise capacity. Most patients who require supplemental oxygen before they begin the program continue to require oxygen afterward. However, if the oxygen is being used as a response to a recent infection or exacerbation of an infection, and if the lung heals from the infection, you may not need oxygen after the rehabilitation program. Also, if you have required only a small amount of supplemental oxygen before the program, there may be a possibility that you can stop oxygen afterward.

83. Is pulmonary rehabilitation covered by my insurance?

It depends. Insurance coverage for pulmonary rehabilitation programs depends on your insurance policy. Even if you have coverage for pulmonary rehabilitation, not all programs may be covered by your policy. It is very important to contact your insurance company or your case manager and ask about your coverage for pulmonary rehabilitation in general, and then ask about coverage for a specific program in your area. Remember, not all pulmonary rehabilitation programs in your area may be covered.

If you do not have a program in your area, or if the program in your area is not covered by insurance, there are many things you can do on your own. Your quality of life can be improved by stopping smoking, learning how to correctly use inhaled medicines, and exercising regularly. Reading books like this can help you learn about your disease and how best to improve your quality of life. When exercising, a simple comfortable plan is best. Choose a place to exercise that is not too hot or too cold, where the air quality is good and it is safe to walk. Some people choose to walk around their neighborhood, some walk in an air-conditioned mall, and others enjoy riding a stationary bicycle in their homes while watching television.

Below is a simple exercise plan for a person with a lung condition. Before starting any exercise program, talk with your health care provider and make sure that this is safe for you to do.

Begin walking slowly at a very comfortable pace for a period of time (say 5–10 minutes daily) 3–5 days a week. Do not increase the time you are walking until you can walk the entire time without stopping. When you can walk without stopping to rest, increase the time you are walking by 1–2 minutes each week. For example, if you can walk nonstop for 5 minutes a day for 5 days in 1 week, increase your walking to 7 minutes each day. Many people with severe lung disease can reach the goal of walking 30 minutes without stopping. Some people with lung problems require oxygen during exercise. If you have been prescribed oxygen for regular use, be sure to use it with exercise. If you are not sure about using oxygen, talk with your health care provider. Some of the resources listed later in this book may help you either find a program or provide you with more information about lung conditions.

Many people with severe lung disease can reach the goal of walking 30 minutes without stopping.

Cecil's comment:

These are my thoughts on extending the life of any patient with COPD. The key to a longer and better life is the will to do it. While I'm not an expert, I have gained knowledge through years of experience. Some of my suggestions are:

Rehabilitation for COPD

1. *Education: it is very important that you educate your-self about COPD and the things you can do to make life easier and prolong your life. Dr. Quinn gives an excellent list of resources at the end of this book. These will give you any information you need and will give you good insight into how to gain control of your illness. If you do not have a computer or computer skills, it would be beneficial to obtain a computer or to learn to use those that are available at most libraries.*

2. *Medical support: If you don't have a primary care physician and a pulmonologist who you can work with and who are willing to work with you, then you need to find them as soon as possible.*

3. *Regardless of the severity of your illness, I would stress that you "hound" your medical support about pulmonary rehabilitation, if you have one in your area and if your insurance will pay for it. This program is probably the most beneficial in enhancing your understanding of your illness and how to control your individual problems.*

4. *Oximeter: You might want to talk to your doctor about the possibility of your insurance company purchasing an oximeter. A sample letter for your doctor to request the oximeter is available at www.olivija.com/lungs/. This will allow you to monitor the oxygen saturation in your blood while you are doing your daily chores and exercising. Oxygen readings below 88% can be dangerous to your other internal organs.*

5. *Smoking: If you are a smoker, then I suggest that you stop ASAP! Cigarettes almost double your deterioration rate with this illness.*

6. *Exercise: This can be a life saver and in most cases will improve your quality of life. I know you are thinking "How do I exercise when I can't breathe?" This can be*

accomplished, and when you get accustomed to it, the ease will surprise you. Pursed-lip breathing is a great help in this area. This is accomplished by breathing in through your nose and counting to four at the same time. Then you forcefully exhale, counting to eight. This is also great for lowering anxiety and pulse rate. Remember, you should always consult your physician before starting any exercise program.

Exercise is so important. If your muscles are toned, more oxygen can flow to your internal organs, where it is most critical. Exercising is also well covered in the first list of sites.

7. *Diet: It is important to control your weight. If you let yourself get too thin, which is a side effect in some cases, you will become too weak to handle all the other areas that need attention. If you become overweight, then you will have extra exertion and a constant strain on your diaphragm, causing shortness of breath.*

7. *Maintain a good mental outlook. If your situation does start to affect your mood, that is, if you become sad or depressed, see a doctor to assess your situation. Medication for depression or anxiety may be required. This is a fairly common side effect of our illness. If a person allows depression to go untreated, then he or she won't be able to address the physical aspects of this illness.*

PART NINE

Surgical Treatment of COPD

Am I a candidate for lung-volume reduction surgery?

Who is a candidate for lung transplantation?

More . . .

84. My doctor has mentioned that my COPD may be improved by lung surgery. What type of surgery is that?

There are several different types of lung surgery that can improve severe COPD: bullectomy, volume reduction surgery, and lung transplantation.

85. What is a bullectomy?

Bullectomy

the surgical removal of bullae in the lung.

A **bullectomy** is the surgical removal of over-inflated air sacs called bullae. These sacs are made up of what remains of hundreds of destroyed air sacs (alveoli). The bullae do not exchange oxygen well and are therefore poorly functioning lung tissue. Unfortunately, these bullae can increase in size and compress parts of the lung that do work well, thus decreasing the overall function of the lung.

In the patient with COPD, a bullectomy helps restore the work of the good parts of the lungs and removes the large, useless air sacs caused by COPD. Most people with COPD have many good sacs available throughout the lungs and therefore would not benefit from surgery, or they may have many bullae in the lung that are small and cannot be surgically removed.

Lung-volume reduction surgery

a type of surgery on the lungs that removes the upper one third of one or both lungs in order to decrease hyperinflation and improve breathing.

86. What is lung–volume reduction surgery?

Lung-volume reduction surgery is an innovative emphysema treatment; it is a surgical procedure in which the most damaged areas lung tissue are removed. Like the surgery for a bullectomy, lung-volume reduction surgery involves removing useless air sacs. However, unlike the bullectomy, lung-volume reduction surgery removes about one third of the upper portion of each lung (the upper lobes). This third of the lung may include some good tissue, but it is mostly useless tissue. This allows the remaining, less diseased, portion of the lung more room to function, resulting in easier breathing. Because it is a major procedure, the circumstances must be just right for it to be performed. This procedure is not a cure, but in selected patients, it can improve breathing, and it provides an alternative to lung transplantation.

87. Am I a candidate for lung-volume reduction surgery?

Lung-volume reduction surgery can reduce hyperinflation of the lungs in patients with COPD. It should be considered in patients with severe upper-lobe emphysema, who have reduced exercise capacity and are not doing well with medical treatment alone. Only people with a lot of emphysema in the upper lungs (seen on a CT scan) benefit. The individual must have a strong heart and a healthy remaining lung after the procedure to justify the risk of the surgery. The patient must also show that he or she is willing to keep physically fit. For this reason, many surgeons require a person to stop smoking and complete a program of pulmonary rehabilitation before having the surgery. The success of this surgery depends on the type of surgery, the severity of the patient's lung and heart disease, and the person's motivation to work to get well after the surgery.

If you and your surgeon agree that this surgery will be beneficial, the following tests are usually ordered:

- Chest x-ray study
- CT scan of chest
- Perfusion scan of lungs
- Blood tests (alpha-1 antitrypsin; cotinine level)
- Complete pulmonary function test with lung volumes by plethysmography
- Room air arterial blood gas
- Dobutamine stress test of heart
- Cardiopulmonary exercise test

After the completion of these tests, the pulmonologist and surgeon then evaluate the interested patient. Jointly, they make the decision as to the candidate's eligibility to proceed with lung-volume reduction surgery. All patients, whether surgical candidates or not, are evaluated and prescribed a pulmonary rehabilitation program by the rehabilitation medical physician during their evaluation at the center.

If a patient is accepted for surgery, he or she is referred to a 6-week outpatient pulmonary rehabilitation program. New techniques may make lung-volume reduction surgery less traumatic and more accessible to selected individuals.

The National Emphysema Therapy Trial, which evaluated lung-volume reduction surgery, has recently reported that surgery was superior to ordinary pulmonary rehabilitation. This means that the patient undergoing this surgery can expect less shortness of breath and better exercise tolerance. A limited number of patients can be freed from the use of long-term oxygen therapy, at least for a period of time

88. What is lung transplantation surgery?

Since the early 1990s, more than 6400 lung transplantations have been performed, and lung transplantation programs exist in many countries. Lung transplantation involves the removal of one or both diseased lungs from the patient with COPD. Currently, single-lung transplantation is preferred to double-lung transplantation for most patients with emphysema because it affords more effective use of a limited supply of donor organs. Lung transplantation is major surgery, and there can be significant complications, including postoperative infection and **rejection** of the new lung by the patient's immune system. Therefore, lung transplantation is available for only a select few patients, and the selection of ideal patients is critical.

Transplant rejection

the rejection by the body's immune system of a foreign tissue or organ.

89. Who is a candidate for lung transplantation?

Patients with end-stage pulmonary disease should be considered for potential lung transplantation if they meet the following criteria:

- Untreatable end-stage pulmonary disease of any etiology
- Absence of other significant medical diseases
- Substantial limitation of daily activities
- Limited life expectancy
- Ambulatory status with rehabilitation potential
- Acceptable nutritional status
- Satisfactory psychosocial profile and emotional support system

Common reasons for unsuitability for a lung transplantation include lung disease that is not severe enough to justify the risk of transplantation, health that is not strong enough to undergo the procedure, or other organs in their body (e.g., heart, liver) that are not functioning properly. Patients with COPD who had any of the following conditions would absolutely not be considered candidates for transplantation:

- Active extrapulmonary infection (pneumonia, tuberculosis, fungal infections)
- Significant disease of other organ systems (e.g., Alzheimer's disease; heart, liver, or kidney disease; or cancer)
- Current cigarette smoking
- Poor nutritional status
- Poor rehabilitation potential
- Significant psychosocial problems, substance abuse, or history of medical noncompliance

90. When should a patient be referred for lung transplantation?

Like all medical treatments, the doctor and patient must weight the risks of the procedure against the possible benefits that will be achieved by it. Patients should be referred for transplantation at a point in the course of their disease at which death is considered likely within several years. The transplantation, in this situation, would be expected to confer a survival advantage to the patient with COPD. If the patient has a particularly poor quality of life because of his or her COPD, this would be an added consideration in the evaluation of the need for a transplantation.

91. What are the outcomes for patients who undergo lung transplantation?

The International Society for Heart and Lung Transplantation and the St. Louis International Lung Transplantation Registry report 1-year survival rates of 71% and 5-year survival rates of 45% after lung transplantation. The commonest causes of mortality after lung transplantation are infection and graft failure or rejection.

According to the registry of the International Society of Heart and Lung Transplantation, 1-, 3-, and 5-year survival rates after lung transplantation are 70.7%, 54.8%, and 42.6%, respectively. The most common survival time is 3.7 years. These rates lag behind those of heart and liver transplantation, for which 5-year survival is approximately 70%.

92. Does lung transplantation increase life expectancy in patients with COPD?

Because candidates for lung transplantation have a short life expectancy and no studies have been preformed to compare similar patients who under versus those who do not undergo transplantation, the answer to this question remains unknown. A survival advantage has been reported for patients with cystic fibrosis and pulmonary fibrosis who have received transplants, but this advantage has not been demonstrated for patients with emphysema.

PART TEN

Nutritional Guidelines for People with COPD

What is the impact of nutrition on immunity?

My doctor says that I'm malnourished.
What should I do?

More . . .

93. Is nutrition a problem with patients with COPD?

Close to three fourths of patients with COPD have significant weight loss. Patients who are malnourished have more lung infections, spend more time in the hospital, and have a shorter life span than those who are well nourished. A recent study of patients with severe COPD who were dependent on oxygen revealed that doctors could predict which of the patients would have more lung infections, respiratory failures, and hospitalizations based on their nutritional status. In this French study, patients who were nutritionally depleted suffered the most. In fact, the best prognosis was observed in overweight and obese patients.

> *Close to three fourths of patients with COPD have significant weight loss.*

94. Why are patients with COPD underweight?

Not all patients with COPD are underweight. However, as patients' symptoms get more severe, they tend to lose weight and muscle mass. Identifying a single cause for this is difficult. Many factors can cause weight loss in COPD, and they can often act in concert. The most significant cause of weight loss for the COPD patient is the extra effort of breathing. The patient with COPD expends so much energy in the simple act of breathing that the ventilatory muscles can require up to 10 times the calories required by a healthy person's muscles. Other common factors include chronic mouth breathing and shortness of breath that make it difficult to chew and swallow, certain medications that can decrease the appetite, and depression.

95. Are underweight COPD sufferers at increased risk?

Malnutrition can worsen symptoms of COPD by decreasing ventilatory muscle strength, exercise tolerance, and immunocompetence, and by increasing the risk of depression and anxiety. Improper nutrition can cause wasting of the diaphragm and other pulmonary muscles. The amount of muscle wasting is worsened if the patient is taking glucocorticosteroids for a long time. (e.g., oral steroids like prednisone or inhaled steroids like **AeroBid**, beclomethasone). When the respiratory muscles get weak, it becomes difficult for the patient to clear mucus out of his lungs, resulting in a need to breathe harder and faster. If this increase in demand escalates, it can lead to respiratory failure. Patients with COPD who are very underweight get sick more often and have a shorter life expectancy than normal weight or even obese patients.

AeroBid
brand name for the medication flunisolide, an inhaled steroid.

96. What is the impact of nutrition on immunity?

A diet deficient in calories, protein, and vitamins and minerals has a negative effect on immune function as well. Poor diet makes it difficult for the body to build new white blood cells and immune factors that are needed to fight infections and to repair damaged tissues. Poor nutrition is common in patients with COPD and puts them at risk for developing respiratory infections. For this reason, the patient with COPD must achieve a balance of good nutrition and exercise to stay as healthy as possible.

97. My doctor says that I'm malnourished. What should I do?

Your physician can assess your current nutritional status. Your physician may counsel you or refer you to a licensed nutritional counselor. He or she will develop an individualized diet plan for you, with recommendations for intake of fats, carbohydrates, protein, and water. The goals of this plan to improve your nutrition should include

- Prevention or reversal of malnutrition without worsening of the disease process
- Achievement of a desirable body weight
- Improvement in respiratory function
- Reduction in the number of lung infections and visits to the hospital
- Improvement in your quality of life

Surprisingly, the use of oral supplements (like Ensure) to improve nutritional health have not been shown to have long-term benefits. Nutritional studies in patients with COPD have shown that higher caloric intake alone does not appear to reverse the weight loss and malnutrition that occurs in advanced emphysema. Improved nutrition, along with optimized medical treatment and rehabilitation, are recommended.

Try to eat your main meal early. This way, you will have lots of energy to carry you through the day.

If your doctor does not feel that you are underweight or malnourished, it is still important to watch your weight and your diet to prevent this from happening. The American Association for Respiratory Care has gathered some nutrition tips for persons with COPD. These are only general guidelines.

1. Eat foods from each of the basic food groups (like your mother told you to). These include

fruits and vegetables, dairy products, cereal and grains, and proteins.

2. Limit your salt intake. Too much sodium can cause you to retain fluids, which may interfere with breathing.

3. Limit your intake of caffeinated drinks. Caffeine may interfere with some of your medications and may also make you feel nervous.

4. Avoid foods that produce gas or make you feel bloated. The best process to use in eliminating foods from your diet is trial and error.

5. Try to eat your main meal early. This way, you will have lots of energy to carry you through the day.

6. Choose foods that are easy to prepare. Do not waste all of your energy preparing a meal.

7. Avoid foods that supply little or no nutritional value.

8. Try eating six small meals a day instead of three large ones. This will keep you from filling up your stomach and causing shortness of breath.

9. If you are using oxygen, be sure to wear your cannula while eating—and after meals, too. Eating and digestion require energy, and this causes your body to use more oxygen.

10. Try to eat in a relaxed atmosphere, and make your meals attractive and enjoyable.

98. I've been told that anabolic steroids may help me to gain weight. Is that true?

Yes. In other populations, such as in frail elderly, cancer, and HIV patients, **anabolic steroids** have been shown to increase a patient's weight. According to a new study, older, malnourished men with COPD benefited from the same type of controversial drug that

Anabolic steroid

a steroid compound with the ability to increase muscle mass.

athletes sometimes use to increase muscle and enhance performance. When a small group of male patients with COPD, who were underweight, were treated for 8 weeks with anabolic steroids, the men experienced weight gain and increases in their muscle mass. The study was reported in *CHEST*, the journal of the American College of Chest Physicians. However, the authors noted that although their patients increased their weight, they did not appear to have an increase in their ability to exercise. Because this study only lasted 8 weeks, it is unknown whether this weight gain will result in decreased episodes of illness or increased life expectancy. More studies with anabolic steroids are planned.

99. Is alternative or complementary medicine helpful in COPD?

Alternative medicine and complimentary medicine are terms that are often used interchangeably and are used as such in this text.

Alternative medicine is a mixed group of practices that include the areas of hygiene, diagnosis, and treatment of many diseases.

Alternative medicine is a mixed group of practices that include the areas of hygiene, diagnosis, and treatment of many diseases. The theoretical bases of alternative medicine diverge from those of modern scientific medicine and are not generally accepted by modern physicians. Alternative medicine has failed to gain acceptance because these practices currently lack a plausible scientific basis or studies demonstrating their safety and efficacy.

Alternative medicine may come from some of the following sources:

- Religious
- Cultural

- Supernatural, magical, or cultist
- Naive, illogical, or false understandings of anatomy, physiology, pathology, or pharmacology
- Fraud and exploitation of the sick and hopeless

Any treatment that is outside the traditional medicine or practice of your primary health system can be considered alternative medicine. A treatment that is alternative in one culture may be traditional in another. For example, acupuncture is a system of treatment that has been practiced in China for more than 5000 years, yet in the United States, it is considered an alternative medicine.

Practitioners of Western (allopathic) medicine are closely monitored and regulated in the United States, having to undergo rigorous training and testing as well as licensing by state and federal authorities. The facilities of modern practitioners, such as hospitals, surgical centers, and dialysis units, undergo similar scrutiny and licensing. Complementary medicines practitioners and their therapies are rarely, if ever, subject to this level of testing and regulation in the United States. Therefore, patients who seek these therapies cannot be confident in the abilities of the practitioners to safely practice their remedies.

The greatest risk involved with using complementary medicine is missing a necessary or possibly life-saving diagnosis or treatment from a practitioner of conventional medicine. It is always best to get as much information as possible—on both complementary and conventional treatments—and then make an informed decision in your consultation with your primary health professional.

Other risks associated with complementary therapies include the potential for dangerous interactions with conventional therapies, a lack of evidence on the effectiveness of many complementary therapies, and the fact that the expense of many complementary therapies may not be covered by health insurance.

The growing consumer interest in alternative medicine has expanded the market for a wide range of products, from acupuncture to the multiple dietary supplements, which are now on the market. Supplements are popular, but are they safe?

Since 1994, when Congress decided that dietary supplements would be regulated as if they were foods, they are assumed to be safe unless the FDA could demonstrate that they pose a significant risk to the consumer. Manufacturers are not legally required to provide specific information about safety before marketing their products. Further, some supplements may interfere with your other COPD medications. Therefore, supplements should be used with caution and only after discussions with your treating physician.

The following are some alternative medicine treatments you may want to discuss with your physician:

- *Acupuncture:* Acupuncture has been shown to decrease breathlessness, increase walking distance, and improve lung function in COPD. Acupuncture may also help patients quit smoking.
- *Herbs.*
  - Ephedra and ma-huang have commonly been used for bronchitis, asthma, and emphysema because of their bronchodilating effect. Because

of the availability of prescription bronchodilators that are standardized, safer, and more effective, the use of ephedra is no longer appropriate.

- *Mullein* is often recommended for cough and bronchitis because of its expectorant effect.

- *Ginseng:* Ginseng is a root that has been used to treat patients with various illnesses for the past 2000 years, particularly in Asian cultures. In a recent study of patients with moderately severe COPD published in *Alternative Medicine Review*, when compared to patients given placebos (sugar pills), patients treated with ginseng for 3 months had measurable improvement in their PFTs and exercise capacity. No side effects were observed.

- *Antioxidants:* Antioxidants, such as vitamins C and E, may help reduce oxidative damage that occurs during flare-ups of emphysema and have both been shown to prevent the oxidative damage caused by exposure to smoke and air pollution. Further, elevated levels of vitamin C seem to be associated with a lower incidence of bronchitis. Although elevated dietary levels of vitamin E and beta carotene are associated with a decreased incidence of chronic bronchitis, studies using vitamin E and beta carotene to prevent bronchitis have had only mixed results.

- *Essential fatty acids:* Fatty acids are the building materials of fats. Most fatty acids can be produced in your body; however, the essential fatty acids need to be part of your diet because they cannot be produced by your body. There are two essential fatty acids: alpha linolenic acid and linoleic acid. Alpha linolenic acid, also known as the omega 3 fatty acid, is found in flax seed, walnuts, and canola oil. Linoleic acid, also known as omega 6 fatty acid, is found in soy, sunflower seeds, and corn oil and most nuts. Essential fatty acids tend to be low in patients with emphysema, who also have low immunity. The essential fatty acids in fish oil may reduce airway irritability and help with a variety of chronic lung diseases.

- *Aromatherapy:* Aromatherapy may be of some benefit in patients with emphysema, but more convincing research is needed.
- *Biofeedback:* Biofeedback has been used to reduces stress and relieve anxiety in many studies. Research in its use in COPD is lacking.
- *Yoga:* Most people who try yoga find that it increases flexibility and reduces stress. Studies have also shown that yoga can help people who have asthma and COPD learn to breathe more easily.
- *Ionized air:* Ionized air has been recommended for patients with chronic lung disease; however, this recommendation is based on very limited research. More research is needed to substantiate this claim.
- *Exercise:* Exercise has been repeatedly been shown to improve quality of life, endurance, and lung function in patients with emphysema—especially when combined with inspiratory muscle training. This is covered more fully in the section on pulmonary rehabilitation.
- *Massage:* In a single, very small study, massage therapy was associated with measurable improvements in lung function in patients with COPD. More research is needed to substantiate this claim.

Before you try any of these therapies, discuss their possible benefits and side effects with your health professional. Let him or her know if you are already using any such therapies.

Cecil's comment:

I am going to close this book by saying that it all seems scary and complicated, and you are probably wondering what you are into at this time. I can say I have known people who have lived for years with this illness and are now in their 70s and 80s. A lot depends on the individual. When you become familiar with all of this and get a daily routine established, it is not much different from anything else. Below are some tips received from a friend of mine who has done remarkably well in regaining control of her illness and seems to be doing exceptionally well.

A person does not realize how important it is to get themselves into a regular daily routine of bedrest. I was instructed to sleep at least 6 hours per night. I have finally gotten to the point where I get between 8 and 9 hours of sleep per night. It also is important to get your medications in a routine. Using a written schedule and pill organizers help some people.

For the ones who are very short of breath, please keep moving the best you can. Exercise is a necessity, even if it is taking only one step. Consider it an accomplishment. Keep a daily record so you can look at it at the end of a week and say I did accomplish this!! Each step forward means a lot!!! I'll close on this note!! Each step means that step FORWARD, I can't express that enough!!! Attitude is everything.

> *Before you try any of these therapies, discuss their possible benefits and side effects with your health professional.*

100. Where can I go for more information?

There are many organizations and publications that can provide you with more information. A list of many such resources is provided in the Appendix.

Appendix

Organizations

COPD International

http://www.copd-international.com/

Your international support network. A web site containing information, resources and discussion forums about COPD.

The American Lung Association

http://www.lungusa.org

This site provides a wide array of information about COPD as well as other lung diseases. The information includes health statistics, risk factors, treatment options, research studies, publications related to lung disease, local programs and events, and links to other lung-related sites.

National Heart, Lung, and Blood Institute (NHLBI)

www.nhlbi.nih.gov/health/public/lung/ www.nhlbi.nih.gov/health/dci/ Diseases/Copd/Copd_WhatIs.html

www.nhlbi.nih.gov/health/public/lung/other/copd_fact.htm

http://www.nhlbi.nih.gov/

This site provides detailed medical information and patient education pamphlets that can be printed out. It also provides information about current treatment and on-going research. There are numerous links to other sites that might be useful for people with COPD as well as other heart and lung diseases.

National Heart, Lung, and Blood Institute

By Telephone: 301-251-1222
By mail: National Heart, Lung, and Blood Institute
P.O. Box 30105
Bethesda, MD 20824-0105

American College of Chest Physicians

http://www.chestnet.org

The American College of Chest Physicians (ACCP) is a medical specialty society of physicians, surgeons, allied health professionals, and individuals with PhD degrees who specialize in diseases of the chest: pulmonology, cardiology, cardiovascular and cardiothoracic surgery, hypertension, critical care medicine, and related disciplines.

This site provides medical information, up-to-date medical alerts regarding medications used to treat lung diseases, and links to patient support groups and other informative sites.

American Association for Respiratory Care (AARC)

http://www.aarc.org

AARC's mission is to advance the science, technology, ethics, and art of respiratory care through research and education for its members and to teach the general public about pulmonary lung health and disease prevention.

This site provides detailed patient education information about COPD and its treatment, including nutritional therapies, safe exercise, reduction of the symptoms of COPD, and use of supplemental oxygen. There is also information on how to get help to quit smoking or to reduce indoor air pollution and links to other lung-related health and patient-oriented sites.

The American Lung Association

www.lungusa.org

The American Lung Association is the oldest voluntary health organization in the United States, with a national office and chapters around the country.

National Emphysema/COPD Association (NECA)

www.necacommunity.org

The NECA is a patient-centered, member-driven, and member-governed organization. Its mission is to empower patients, families, and caregivers to improve the quality of patient care and the quality of their lives.

National Emphysema Foundation (NEF)

http://emphysemafoundation.org/

By Telephone: 203-849-9000

By Fax: 203-286-1105

By Mail: NEF

15 Belden Avenue

Norwalk, CT 06850

The NEF was founded in 1971; its mission is to improve the quality of life of patients with emphysema, asthma, or related lung diseases with information and education for families. The NEF supports research and works with many advisors who are involved in direct patient care.

The information presented here is from experienced professionals, and they have written their expert opinions specifically for the web site. Information is also presented from published literature.

Centers for Disease Control and Prevention: Facts About Chronic Obstructive Pulmonary Disease (COPD)

www.cdc.gov/nceh/airpollution/copd/copdfaq.htm

The Centers for Disease Control and Prevention (CDC) is recognized as the leading federal agency for protecting the health and safety of people—at home and abroad, providing credible information to enhance health decisions and promoting health through strong partnerships.

National Lung Health Education Program (NLHEP)

www.nlhep.org

The prevention of lung disease and the promotion of lung health is the goal of the NLHEP, conducted in collaboration with government, medical, and other health professional organizations.

Appendix

153

Web Sites for Patients

HealthyResources

http://www.healthyresources.com/copd/

HealthyResources for managing COPD provides books (*Courage and Information*), information (*COPD TODAY*, an on-line magazine), community, services, and products to help you (and your family) to manage your health. Patients collaborate with health care professionals to empower people with COPD and their families.

Chronic Lung Disease (CLD) Forum

http://www.cheshire-med.com/programs/pulrehab/forum/ cldforum.html

Patients with CLD, as well as their families and friends, are invited to share their questions, experiences, discoveries, and support. We offer a number of ways to communicate with and assist the members of our community of caring. Sponsored by the Cheshire Medical Center, the CLD forum provides information and a on-line forum to discussion of issues related to chronic lung disease.

Centers for Disease Control and Prevention, COPD FASTATS

www.cdc.gov/nchs/fastats/copd.htm

National Institutes of Health: COPD Health Information

health.nih.gov/result.asp?disease_id=165

Medline Plus: COPD Health Information

www.nlm.nih.gov/medlineplus/copdchronicobstructivepulmonary disease.html

COPD—Alert

www.copd-alert.com

COPD—Alert is a support and advocacy web site.

Global Initiative for Chronic Obstructive Lung Disease (GOLD)

www.goldcopd.com

GOLD provides the latest medical consensus on the diagnosis and treatment of COPD.

ibreathe.com

ibreathe.com

Glaxo-Smith Kline, a pharmaceutical company, has sponsored a
web site that offers information for people with respiratory
conditions and their caregivers about COPD and smoking cessation.

Emphysema Foundation for Our Right to Survive

www.emphysema.net

This foundation provides on-line information and resources and
a listserv for support. It is a nonprofit organization of patients
and family caregivers.

Web Resources for Caregivers

Caregiver.com

http://www.caregiver.com

Caregiver.com contains back issues of Today's Caregiver Magazine, information on "Sharing Wisdom Caregivers Confer-
ences," and a discussion forum.

Caregiver Resource Directory

Offered by Beth Israel Medical Center, this practical guide is
intended to help family caregivers feel less alone and over-
whelmed. It offers resources, facts, and advice about caring for
a loved one, as well as offering help for the caregiver. The
Directory is designed as an interactive three-ring binder with
pockets and ample writing space so that caregivers can organize
all resource and medical information in one place. The Directory can be ordered on-line at *http://stoppain.org/caregivers/
resource_form.html.*

CareGuide

http://www.careguide.com

CareGuide provides resources for family caregivers. It includes
everything they need to assess, plan, manage, and monitor the
best care for their loved ones.

COPD-Support, Inc.

http://www.copd-support.com

COPD-Support, Inc. is a nonprofit corporation that provides a means of communication in order to provide support and education for individuals who have COPD, for their caregivers and for others who have an interest in the disease.

Family Caregiver Alliance

http://www.caregiver.org/

This organization has provided more than 20 years of advocacy and support for family caregivers. The site features on-line support for family caregivers, as well as bilingual information for Spanish-speaking people.

Friends' Health Connection

http://www.48friend.com

This group links caregivers of people with disabilities and chronic illness. It also has links to caregiver support organizations.

National COPD Coalition

www.uscopd.com

The National COPD Coalition brings together heath professional organizations, patient organizations and foundations, individuals, and government agencies to improve the lives of people with COPD.

American Association for Respiratory Care (AARC)

The AARC is a professional membership association for respiratory therapists. Respiratory therapists assist in the diagnosis and treatment of patients with pulmonary disorders. The AARC provides educational programs to the respiratory care community and promotes the art and science of respiratory care to health care consumers and other health care professionals.

American College of Chest Physicians

http://www.chestnet.org/

Their mission is to promote the prevention and treatment of diseases of the chest through leadership, education, research, and communication. The ACCP has nearly 15,000 members in more 100 countries worldwide who specialize in various multidisciplinary areas of chest medicine. The ACCP meets its mission and vision by providing physicians, researchers, and health-care practitioners with such resources as continuing education courses and products; *CHEST, The Cardiopulmonary and Critical Care Journal*, and other publications; consensus statements and clinical practice guidelines; representation in government public affairs; The CHEST Foundation; and a myriad of other resources.

Resources for Smoking Cessation

The Centers for Disease Control and Prevention (CDC)
http://www.cdc.gov/tobacco/how2quit.htm
The CDC provides information and resources on quitting smoking.

The US Department of Health and Human Services
http://www.surgeongeneral.gov/tobacco/
This government office offers a Tobacco Cessation Guideline, including the latest drugs and counseling techniques for treating tobacco use and dependence.

The American Lung Association
http://www.lungusa.org/site/pp.asp?c=dvLUK9O0E&b=44456
The American Lung Association provides a smoking cessation resource fact sheet.

QuitNet
http://www.quitnet.com/
QuitNet is an on-line resource for information and forums on quitting smoking.

RESOURCES FOR Alpha1 Antitrypsin Disease
http://www.NationalJewish.org/medfacts/alpha1.html
The National Jewish Medical and Research Center is one of the leading centers in the nation for the study of lung disease.

The Alpha-1 Association
www.alpha1.org
The Alpha-1 Association is nonprofit organization run for and by people suffering from alpha 1 antitrypsin deficiency and is focused on education, awareness, patient protection and advocacy.

The Alpha-1 Foundation

www.alphaone.org

The Alpha-1 Foundation is another great nonprofit organization whose focus is mainly directed toward the needs of doctors, clinicians, researchers, and the like. This is a great place to find a good doctor or center of excellence for alpha-1 antitrypsin deficiency.

The dailylung.com Guide to Alpha-1-Antitrypsin Deficiency

www.dailylung.org/aat.htm/

The Daily Lung is a good resource of understandable information.

Alpha-1 Research Registry

www.alphoneregistery.org

The Alpha-1 Research Registry consists of individuals with alpha-1 antitrypsin deficiency or a carrier phenotype who are willing to participate in research to promote the development of improved treatments and a cure.

Clinical Trials

Before an investigational drug or treatment can be considered for approval by the US Food and Drug Administration (FDA), it must be shown to be both safe and effective. Typically, this is accomplished via clinical research trials—carefully designed and monitored studies intended to test and evaluate investigational drugs and treatment plans.

People may be interested in clinical trials for a variety of reasons. Some people participate in clinical trials as a way to contribute to medical science and to help doctors and researchers find better ways to help others. Others participate in clinical trials to receive investigational treatments because their illness is not responding to standard treatment. Their hope is that the study treatment—possibly an investigational drug or a combination of drugs—will work better for them than standard therapy. If you are interested in participating in a clinical trial for patients with COPD, go to *www.acecopdtrial.com*

Other Books Worth Reading About COPD

Petty TL (Foreword), Shimberg EF. Coping with COPD: Understanding, Treating, and Living with Chronic Obstructive Pulmonary Disease. St. Martin's Griffin, New York, NY 2003.

Carter R et al. Courage and Information for Life with Chronic Obstructive Pulmonary Disease: The Handbook for Patients, Families and Care Givers Managing COPD, Emphysema, Bronchitis. New Technology Publishing; 2nd edition (September 1, 2001) Onset, MA.

Schachter N. Life and Breath: Preventing, Treating and Reversing Chronic Obstructive Pulmonary Disease. Broadway; 1st edition (April 8, 2003).

Haas F, Sperber Haas S. The Chronic Bronchitis and Emphysema Handbook. Wiley; 1st edition (October 15, 2000).

Adams FV. The Breathing Disorders Sourcebook. McGraw-Hill; 1 edition (November 1, 1998).

Barnes PJ et al. Asthma and COPD: Basic Mechanisms and Clinical Management. Academic Press; 1st edition (May, 2002).

Appendix

Glossary

Arterial blood gas (ABG): A measure of the oxygen and carbon dioxide in the bloodstream. The ABG is measured from a sample of blood removed from an artery, usually in the wrist or elbow.

AccuNeb: A bronchodilator. A brand name for the medication albuterol sulfate.

N-Acetylcysteine: A type of medicine that may help move secretions out of the lungs and airways. A brand name is Mucomyst.

Action plan: A written document that gives specific instructions on what to do if you feel you need to see a doctor in an emergency.

Adrenal suppression: A decrease in the body's production of adrenal steroids as a result of taking medications that contain these steroids, such as prednisone or hydrocortisone.

Advanced directive: A general term that refers to your oral and written instructions about your future medical care, in the event that you become unable to speak for yourself. There are two types of advance directives: a living will and a medical power of attorney.

AeroBid: An inhaled steroid. A brand name for the medication flunisolide.

Agonist: Medicines that exert their affects by combining with places called "receptor sites" on body tissues. Albuterol, for example, attaches to the lungs' beta receptors. Albuterol then is called a "beta agonist." When albuterol attaches to these receptors, it causes the bronchi to dilate (bronchodilation).

Air sac: Also known as an alveolus. It is the space at the end of the smallest airway in the lung. This is the place in the body where inhaled oxygen attaches to the red blood cell and carbon dioxide is released, to be breathed out.

Albuterol sulfate: A short-acting beta agonist bronchodilator. Some brand names are AccuNeb, Proventil, Ventolin, Volmax, and VoSpire.

Alupent: An inhaled bronchodilator of the beta agonist group. A brand name for the medication metaproterenol sulfate.

Alveoli: The small air sacs in the lung where oxygen is exchanged for carbon dioxide in the lung.

Anabolic steroid: A steroid compound with the ability to increase muscle mass. It can be used to treat patients with muscle wasting due to malnourishment. It can be also be used as an illegal performance enhancer by professional athletes.

Antibiotics: A medication, usually derived from a mold or bacterium, that inhibits the growth of other microorganisms. Antibiotics are used to treat infections by bacteria, such as pneumonia.

Anticholinergic agents: A type of medication used as a bronchodilator in patients with COPD. Not a beta agonist.

Asthma: An inflammatory disease of the lung that results in reversible airway obstruction. Unlike COPD, asthma's symptoms tend to wax and wane in severity.

Atrovent: The brand name for ipratropium bromide, an anticholinergic type of bronchodilator.

Beta-agonist medication: A type of medication used as a bronchodilator in patients with COPD. Not an anticholinergic agent.

Bronchi: The main wind pipe divides into to these smaller airways in the middle of the chest.

Bronchiectasis: A chronic dilation of the airways in the lung as the result of chronic inflammation. This condition is often associated with infections and increased sputum production.

Bronchiole: One of the smallest airways in the lung, near the alveoli.

Bronchitis: An inflammation of the bronchi, or small airways, in the lung. It is characterized by cough and sputum production.

Bronchoconstriction: A narrowing of the breathing tubes in the lung. This is the cause of "wheezing."

Bronchodilator: A medication that increases the caliber of the airways of the lungs and makes it easier to breathe.

Bronchospasm A contraction of the smooth muscle in the airways that results in narrower air passages and difficulty breathing. A common condition in people with asthma. It may also be present in lesser amounts in patients with COPD.

Bulla (bullae): Large, thin-walled air sacs in the lung, composed of the remains of many disrupted and distended smaller air sacs.

Bullectomy: The surgical removal of bullae in the lung.

CDC: Center for Disease Control. A division of the National Institute of Health.

Chronic bronchitis: A chronic disease characterized by coughing and sputum production that last for at least 3 months in 2 consecutive years.

Combivent: A combination of two bronchodilators. The medication includes albuterol sulfate and ipratropium bromide that is provided in a metered-dose inhaler and as an inhalation solution to be use with a nebulizer.

Chronic obstructive pulmonary disease (COPD): Several different lung diseases that share similar symptoms and demonstrate a similar pattern of dysfunction shown on spirometry. COPD includes emphysema and chronic bronchitis.

Cor pulmonale: Acute strain or hypertrophy of the right ventricle caused by a disorder of the lungs or of the pulmonary blood vessels.

Corticosteroids: Hormones that are naturally produced by the adrenal glands of your body. They are used therapeutically to mimic or augment the effects of the naturally occurring corticosteroids. Corticosteroids are very powerful drugs that affect the entire body; inhaled corticosteroids or even corticosteroids used on large areas of skin for long periods are absorbed in sufficient quantity to cause systemic effects. They play a role in the immune function as well as the regulation of blood pressure and water balance. *See also:* cortisol.

Cortisol: A steroid produced in the adrenal glands of the body. It helps with suppressing immune function in the body. *See also:* corticosteroids.

Cystic fibrosis: Genetic disorder that affects the lungs. The lining of the lungs produces excess mucus. This mucus clogs the small breathing passages, making it difficult to breathe.

Desaturation: A decrease in the amount of oxygen in the blood.

Diaphragmatic breathing: A type of breathing where the patient uses the diaphragm muscle rather than the chest muscles to breath in an out.

Diffusion capacity: A test used to determine how well oxygen passes from the air sacs of the lungs into the blood. Also known as lung diffusion testing.

Dyspnea: Shortness of breath, a subjective feeling of difficultly or distress in breathing.

Emphysema: A disease of the lungs that causes severe shortness of breath. Emphysema occurs when the walls between the alveoli or air sacs within the lung lose their ability to stretch and recoil. The air sacs become weakened and break. Elasticity of the lung tissue is lost, causing air to be trapped in the air sacs and impairing the exchange of oxygen and carbon dioxide. Also, the support of the airways is lost, allowing for air-flow obstruction.

Endotracheal tube: A flexible tube that is inserted nasally or orally or into a tracheostomy to pump air into the lungs.

Exacerbation: An increase in the severity of the signs or symptoms of a disease.

Expectorant: A medication that helps one to cough up phlegm or mucus.

Expiration: The act of breathing out, or exhaling.

Forced expiratory volume: An important measure of pulmonary function. It is the volume of air that can be forced out of the lungs after taking a deep breath. The forced expiratory volume in the first second is the FEV1.

Forced expiratory volume after 1 second (FEV1): A common spirometric measurement of the volume of air that can be breathed out in 1 second. FEV1 is usually lower in obstructive airways because of mucus secretion, bronchospasm, inflammation, or loss of elastic support of the airways themselves, as in emphysema.

Forced vital capacity (FVC): The maximum volume of gas that can be forcefully and rapidly expired after a maximal inspiration. This maneuver may also be called a "flow-volume loop." Significance: May be normal or reduced in emphysema because of loss of support for small airways.

Formoterol: A long-acting beta agonist that should not be used as a rescue medication. Brand name is Foradil.

Gas diffusion test: Used to determine how well oxygen and other gases pass from the air sacs of the lungs into the blood.

Gastroesophageal reflux disease (GERD): A condition that occurs when acid in the stomach enters the esophagus. It is the cause of "heart burn" or "agita."

Guaifenesin: Medication used to help clear mucus or phlegm from the chest. It works by thinning the mucus or phlegm in the lungs.

HEPA filters: HEPA stands for High Efficiency Particulate Air. It is a type of air filter that removes even very small particles from the air.

Hyperinflation: A condition of the lungs in which the air sacs in the lungs lose their elasticity or stretchiness. When they are inflated during inhalation, they are unable to push out the air, so air is trapped in the lungs.

Hypoxemia: A low oxygen content in the blood stream.

Influenza: An acute infectious respiratory disease caused by the influenza virus. It is characterized by fever, headache, muscle aches, and cough. It usually lasts 3–4 days.

Inspiration: The act of taking in a breath; breathing in.

Ipratropium bromide: An inhaled, short-acting, anticholinergic bronchodilator. Brand name is Atrovent.

Levalbuterol: A type of albuterol sulfate that is formulated to have fewer side effects, such as tremors and rapid heart beats.

Living will: A type of advance directive in which you put in writing your wishes about medical treatment should you be unable to communicate at the end of life.

Lungs: The primary respiratory organs in the chest. Responsible for getting oxygen into the bloodstream and removing carbon dioxide.

Lung-volume reduction surgery: A type of surgery on the lungs that removes the upper one third of one or both lungs in order to decrease hyperinflation and improve breathing.

Metered-dose inhaler (MDI): An aerosol container that dispenses a fixed amount of medication for inhalation. Also called a "puffer."

Medical power of attorney: A document that enables you to appoint someone you trust to make decisions about your medical care if you cannot make those decisions yourself. It is also known as a "health care proxy" or "appointment of a health care agent."

Mucolytic agent: Mucolytic agents are designed to help loosen and clear the mucus from the airways by breaking it up.

Mucus: A clear, sticky mixture composed of water, proteins, and salts secreted by the mucus glands in the nose, sinuses, and airways of the lung.

Nebulizer: A device that changes a liquid respiratory medication into a fine mist that can be inhaled.

Oxygen therapy: A treatment in which an increased concentration of oxygen is made available for breathing, through a nasal catheter, tent, chamber or mask.

Phlegm: Abnormal amounts of mucus, especially as expectorated from the mouth. Often a sign of inflammation or infection.

Pneumococcus vaccination: A compound that induces an immune response. It is used to prevent or decrease the effects of infections from pneumococcus bacteria.

Pneumonia: An infection of one or both lungs that is usually caused by a bacterium, virus, or fungus. Patients with COPD are at increased risk for pneumonia.

Pneumothorax: A condition in which air gets between your lungs and your chest wall. Normally, two thin layers of moist tissue (pleurae) separate the lung and chest wall. Any air that leaks into this space (pleural space) causes the lung tissue to collapse in proportion to the amount of air that enters the pleural cavity.

Polycythemia: An increase above normal in the number of red cells in the blood.

Proventil: A short-acting inhaled bronchodilator A brand name for the medication albuterol sulfate.

Pulmonary fibrosis: A disease of the lungs in which normal lung tissue is replaced with fibroctic (or scar) tissue. When the scar forms, the lung tissue becomes thicker and less able to transfer oxygen into the bloodstream. This process is irreversible.

Pulmonary function tests (PFTs): Tests of lung function that include measurements of lung volumes, breathing capacity, and gas diffusion.

Pulmonologist: A medical specialist in lung diseases.

Pulse oximetry: Noninvasive measure of oxygen saturation, i.e., the amount of oxygen in the bloodstream, recorded in terms of a percentage. This is not as accurate as the values obtained from an ABG and should be used only as a gauge of the amount of oxygen in the blood. Normal ranges are between 95% and 100%. Supplemental oxygen is not generally instituted unless oxygen saturation is less than 88%–90% at rest.

Pursed-lip breathing: A breathing technique used to decrease shortness of breath. Patients with COPD are taught to breathe in through their nose, and then on expiration pucker their lips together as though whistling (this provides back pressure and breathe out slowly through their pursed lips) which keeps the alveoli from collapsing before the end of the breath.

Respirator: A mechanical device that forces air into the lungs of people with respiratory failure. The terms respirator and ventilator are used interchangeably.

Respiratory distress: Difficulty breathing, visibly labored breathing.

Respiratory failure: The inability of your lungs to keep up.

Respiratory therapist: A professional charged with administering any of the therapies related to the respiratory system or breathing.

Salmeterol: An inhaled, long-acting, beta agonist bronchodilator. *Brand name:* Serevent.

Sleep apnea: A condition where the patient has episodes of not breathing during sleep. These episodes can last several seconds to half a minute.

Spacer device: A mechanism to increase the efficiency of inhaled medications. The device is composed of a large plastic container, usually in two halves that click together. At one end is a mouthpiece and at the other end is a hole for inserting the mouthpiece of an MDI (metered-dose inhaler). The dose from your inhaler is sprayed into the spacer, from which it can be inhaled without needing to coordinate breathing and push down the inhaler canister.

Spirometry: A method of making lung function measurements using a device called a spirometer.

Sputum: Expectorated matter, especially mucus expectorated during diseases of the lung.

Steroid: A general name for an anti-inflammatory hormone produced by the adrenal glands.

Theo-Dur: A brand of long-acting theophylline.

Theolair-24®: A brand of long-acting theophylline.

Theophylline: An alkaloid type of medication similar to caffeine that can cause bronchodilation as well as increased respiratory muscle contraction and endurance. Not given often because of its significant side effects.

Thrush: Thrush, a possible side effect of using inhaled steroids, is a yeast infection of the throat that causes white spots or a white layer on the tongue or throat

Tiotropium: A long-acting, inhaled, anticholinergic medication. *Brand name:* Spiriva.

Total lung volume: The amount of air that is contained in the lungs after a deep inspiration.

Trachea: The wind pipe or main airway that goes from the throat to the center of the chest.

Tracheostomy: An operation to make an opening into the main wind pipe in your neck (the trachea).

Transplant rejection: The rejection by the body's immune system of a foreign tissue or organ. Transplant rejection can be diminished or eliminated by immunosuppressive therapy, like steroid medications.

Uni-Dur: A brand of long-acting theophylline

Vaccine: A specialized preparation designed to stimulate the body's system to make protective antibodies directed against specific bacteria or viruses. Some examples are the influenza vaccine and the pneumococcus vaccine.

Ventilator: A mechanical device for forcing air into the lungs of patients with respiratory failure. The terms ventilator and respirator are used interchangeably.

Ventolin: A short-acting inhaled bronchodilator, also known albuterol sulfate.

Wheeze: An abnormal lung sound associated with lung congestion. It is produced when air travels in and out of a narrowed breathing tube that is constricted with inflammation, or accumulated mucus, or both.

Xopenex: A short-acting inhaled bronchodilator A brand name for the medication levalbuterol.

Index